From
Blocked
to
Powerful

The Spiritual Guide to Unlocking
Inner Clarity and Authentic Power

CHERYL STELTE

Copyright © 2024 Cheryl Stelte

All rights reserved.

ISBN: 9798335306195

DEDICATION

To all the incredible souls I've had the honor to guide, and to those I have yet to meet on this journey. Your courage in transformation, uncovering your profound truths, and embracing inner power continually inspires me. May this book be a beacon of light, reflecting the beauty and greatness within you.

Table of Contents

Chapter 1 Introduction 1

Chapter 2 Understanding Subconscious Blocks   7

Chapter 3 Authentic Power 14

Chapter 4 Embracing Discovery and Change . . 22

Chapter 5 From Blocked to Clarity to Purpose (the first time) 34

Chapter 6 First Step to Becoming Your Own Energy Worker 43

Chapter 7 Accessing and Clearing Subconscious Blocks 54

Chapter 8 Empowerment - Reprogramming the Subconscious 68

Chapter 9 Developing Receptivity 76

Chapter 10 Are You a Hole Filler? 88

Chapter 11 New Beginnings 96

Chapter 12 Healing and Empowerment to True Purpose 108

Chapter 13	Spike of Purpose	119
Chapter 14	Clearing Blocks in Your Environment	131
Chapter 15	Evolving Through Heart Centered Shamanism	143
Chapter 16	Take Your Seat	154
Chapter 17	Use Your Struggles to Catapult to a Higher State of Being	167
Chapter 18	From Blocked to Powerful - Summary	181
Chapter 19	Thank You	187

ACKNOWLEDGMENTS

It is with deep appreciation and reverence that I acknowledge the extraordinary spiritual teachers and healers who have guided, inspired, and supported me on my journey. Your wisdom, compassion, and dedication have profoundly shaped my path and allowed me to become the person I am today. Without your guidance, this book—and my life's work—would not have been possible.

First and foremost, I extend my heartfelt gratitude to the late Claude Poncelet. You humbly led by example, teaching us to become our own teachers. Your profound insights and dedication to the evolution of humanity have been a cornerstone of my spiritual growth. Your teachings have illuminated my path and helped me navigate through both the darkness and light of my journey.

To Kathy de Bucy, thank you for your healing hands and open heart. Your energy and guidance have been a source of immense strength and comfort. Your ability to heal and transform has been a true blessing in my life.

I am deeply grateful to Denise Linn, whose wisdom and teachings have provided me with the tools to clear my subconscious blocks and discover clarity. Your teachings have not only empowered me but also enabled me to empower others. Your impact on my journey is immeasurable, and I am forever thankful for your presence.

To Aziza and Jai, your spiritual guidance has been a beacon of light in my life. Your mentorship has been invaluable, and your belief in my potential has been a driving force in my personal and professional growth.

A special thanks to Dr. Usha, India, whose transformational work has inspired me to reach new heights. Your dedication to the healing arts and your ability to facilitate profound change have deeply influenced my approach to healing and empowerment.

I would also like to acknowledge all the wonderful souls not mentioned here who have been a guiding light, helping me to align with my soul's purpose and to help others do the same.

Lastly, to all the unnamed teachers, healers, and spiritual guides who have touched my life in countless ways, I extend my deepest gratitude. Each of you has played a vital role in my journey, and your influence is woven into the fabric of my work. Your contributions have not only enriched my life but have also enabled me to help others on their paths to transformation and clarity.

May this book be a testament to the incredible impact of your teachings and the light you bring into the world. Thank you for being the amazing guiding stars in my journey.

1

Introduction

"We Are All Powerful Beyond Belief, Powerful Beyond What We Can Imagine"

— *Cheryl Stelte*

Welcome to "From Blocked to Powerful: Transform Subconscious Blocks and Discover Clarity for Women Who Know They Are Meant for More." This book is your guide to transforming yourself and your life by removing the hidden barriers that hold you back, uncovering your deepest truths, and stepping into your authentic power.

You might have picked up this book because you feel a strong urge to make changes in your career, business, or life. Perhaps you're seeking more meaning after retirement, or you are clearly aware that you are meant for more, or something better, and are painfully aware of the subconscious blocks that are getting in your way. If so, you're in the right place.

Throughout the pages of this book, you will embark on a journey of, healing, self-discovery, and empowerment. You will learn how to clear your subconscious blocks, find the clarity you've been looking for, and step into your true power to let your greatness shine in your own totally unique way. You can start to live your purpose. Each chapter is designed to provide you with valuable insights and practical techniques to help you navigate this transformative journey.

During my spiritual journey and through various career transitions, I developed a unique approach to helping others. I became an expert in identifying and clearing subconscious blocks, empowering individuals to gain clarity, align with their true purpose, and experience their intentions unfolding. I understand that while there is a wealth of information on setting intentions, many people face frustration when those intentions don't manifest. Linking the manifestation of intentions to the clearing of subconscious blocks is a key concept I've encountered in my work.

Recognizing the power of this approach, I founded the Star of Divine Light Institute and created the Azarias Energy Healing Certification Program. Through these programs, I offer mature women who are so eager for change, from all walks of life, coaches, entrepreneurs, and those men who are committed to transformation, potent tools to catalyze transformative shifts within themselves and those they work with.

My goal is to offer as much as I can within these pages to help you on your journey. I have learned and actively practiced over the years multiple methods and modalities, from healing traditions both modern and ancient and from cultures in various parts of the word . My purpose is to help you experience the ones I have found to be most valuable .

This book is more than just a read; it's a workbook filled with spiritual practices and exercises from an array of spiritual techniques and approaches that will guide you in becoming your own energy worker. You can approach this process in two ways: read or skim through it first to get a sense of the overall journey, then go back and dive into the exercises and techniques; or if you are experiencing an intense longing for transformation or a profound need for change, please, feel that fully and jump right into the healing and empowerment adventure right from the start.

In Chapter 1, "Understanding Subconscious Blocks," you will explore the nature of these hidden barriers that influence your thoughts, emotions, and actions without your conscious awareness. This foundational knowledge is crucial for identifying and addressing the blocks that hinder your personal growth and fulfillment.

In Chapter 2, "Authentic Power," you will delve into the concept of true power, examining how it differs from traditional notions of power and how embracing your authentic power can lead to profound personal transformation. This chapter encourages you to reflect deeply on your relationship with power and helps you align with your higher purpose.

Early on, I share one of my personal stories of clearing blocks, gaining clarity, and living my purpose for the first time. This pivotal moment in my life inspired me to help others embark on their own journeys of self-discovery and empowerment. As you read through the chapters, you will find tools and techniques that have been honed over years of practice, aimed at helping you uncover the hidden blocks that are holding you back, so you can finally step forward into your greatness.

You will explore chapters like "Developing Receptivity" and "Are You a Hole Filler?" which challenge you to look deeper into your behaviors and patterns. Recognizing and understanding these patterns is essential for reprogramming your subconscious and moving toward true empowerment. Remember, this is an ongoing process of growth and self-discovery.

Other chapters, such as "New Beginnings" and "Spike of Purpose," encourage you to embrace change and recognize the moments of clarity that guide you toward your soul's purpose. Every struggle, as highlighted in "Use Your Struggles to Catapult to a Higher State of Being," prepares you with the resilience and wisdom needed to navigate life's challenges and continue your journey toward authentic power.

In chapters like "Evolving Through Heart-Centered Shamanism" and "Take Your Seat," you will learn to see your journey as part of a greater whole. Aligning with your deeper authentic self and your purpose and serving others not only elevates your own life but also contributes to the collective healing and empowerment of those around you.

As you embark on this journey, know that you are not alone. You are now equipped with the knowledge, tools, and confidence to continue your journey with purpose and clarity. Your path is uniquely yours, and every step you take is a testament to your strength and resilience.

If at any point you feel uncertain or need additional support, remember that you don't have to do it all on your own. I am here for you. If it's a quick question, just email me - steltecheryl@gmail.com. If you want more, consider scheduling a discovery call to see if we would be a good fit to work together. gain more personalized insights and guidance. These sessions can help you become aware of the nature of your conscious and subconscious blocks and provide you with the clarity you need to move forward.

You are destined to discover your authentic power. Embrace your journey with an open heart, knowing that every challenge or block is an opportunity for growth and is helping you move forward. Every victory is a stepping stone toward your most powerful, authentic self. As you move forward, let your light shine brightly, inspiring others to embark on their own journeys of healing and empowerment.

Thank you for allowing me to be a part of your transformative journey. Remember, you are powerful beyond belief, powerful beyond what you can currently imagine. You are worthy, you matter so much, you are oh so loveable and you are destined to discover your authentic power.

2

Understanding Subconscious Blocks

"Until you make the unconscious conscious, it will direct your life and you will call it fate."
— *Carl Jung*

Before diving into the transformative steps of personal growth and healing, it's crucial to understand subconscious blocks—those invisible dams that shape our thoughts, emotions, and actions without us even realizing it. These blocks often arise from past traumas, limiting beliefs, or unresolved emotions, and can keep us stuck in unhelpful patterns. By recognizing and addressing these blocks, you can begin to unlock your true potential and move toward a life of greater clarity and empowerment.

Subconscious blocks are unprocessed emotions stored in the right side of your brain. They may stem from past traumas or emotions that influence your thoughts and behaviors without your awareness. These blocks act like invisible chains, hindering your full potential. My goal is to assist you in clearing these blocks, even if their origins are unclear. By clearing these blocks, you'll create space within yourself to access your true self and authentic power hidden by your blocks. You will discover the clarity that already exists within you. The answers you seek are already within; you simply need to open the space to tap into your wisdom.

Subconscious blocks are stored in the right brain as a mix of emotions, physical sensations, and fragmented memories, unlike the linear memories in the left brain. The right brain handles feelings and non-verbal information, so it keeps past experiences that we might not fully understand. These blocks can show up as strong emotions, body discomfort, or bits of memories that seem unclear. Since the right brain doesn't work in a logical, step-by-step way, these blocks can feel jumbled and hard to make sense of. Emotions might feel intense without a clear reason, physical sensations can come up without an obvious cause, and fragmented memories can appear as vivid but incomplete flashes. These stored experiences can affect our actions and feelings, often creating challenges until we recognize and address them.

Imagine trying to move forward while invisible ropes pull you back—these ropes are your subconscious blocks, silently dictating how you respond to life's challenges. Subconscious blocks often arise from past experiences that were painful, distressing, or unresolved at the time you experienced them. When such experiences are intense or traumatic and unresolved, they get imprinted in the right side of the brain, our subconscious mind, creating mental and emotional barriers. Because these blocks operate below our conscious awareness, they can lead us to make choices that don't align with our true desires. For instance, if you have a subconscious block related to fear of failure, you might avoid taking risks or pursuing opportunities, even when you consciously want to.

These blocks influence our behavior subtly but profoundly. They manifest as automatic responses or habits that we fall into without thinking. You might find yourself repeatedly making choices that undermine your goals or happiness, like procrastinating, avoiding challenges, or engaging in negative self-talk. Subconscious blocks often take the form of limiting beliefs—negative thoughts about yourself or the world that hold you back. Moreover, these blocks can trigger automatic emotional responses, such as anxiety, fear, or anger, even when there's no real threat or reason to feel that way. Such emotional reactions can cloud your judgment and prevent you from responding calmly and rationally to situations, often projecting your internal pain onto others.

From a scientific perspective, subconscious blocks can be seen as emotional wounds stored in the subconscious mind. The subconscious mind operates below the level of conscious awareness, storing memories, beliefs, habits, and emotions like a hidden database influencing our conscious thoughts and actions. Emotional wounds are psychological injuries from distressing or traumatic past experiences, stored in the subconscious through neural pathways and connections in the brain, involving areas like the amygdala (which processes emotions) and the hippocampus (which stores memories). These subconscious blocks or emotional wounds can lead to patterns of self-sabotage, fears, and resistance to change. Even when you consciously want to move forward, these blocks can create barriers that make it difficult to progress.

The good news is that the brain has a remarkable ability to change and adapt, known as neuroplasticity. This means it's possible to rewire the neural pathways associated with subconscious blocks. By addressing and healing these emotional wounds, you can gradually release these blocks and experience greater emotional well-being and personal growth. You can actually rewire your brain and overcome these subconscious barriers. As renowned trauma expert Bessel Van Der Kolk emphasizes, trauma isn't just an isolated event; it's an imprint on the mind, brain, and body. By delving beyond the surface-level processes of the mind and addressing the emotional energy trapped within, we can unlock profound and enduring healing.

Trauma isn't just about what happened; it's about what didn't happen. Many of us learned early on that it might not be safe to feel or express our emotions. In some families, emotions were ignored or deemed unacceptable. This emotional neglect is a form of trauma that can be challenging to identify, even for professionals, because it operates silently, hidden beneath the surface. Emotional neglect leaves us with unresolved emotions, resulting in stagnant energy within our systems. This stagnant energy forms patterns that persist throughout our lives. When faced with familiar emotions, we instinctively respond as we did in childhood. Over time, these patterns repeat themselves, leaving us puzzled by the recurrence of similar issues in our relationships, work, or health.

Many highly successful individuals achieve their success driven by a strong desire to overcome past hardships or challenges they've faced. Early life experiences of difficulty, rejection, or adversity often act as powerful motivators, pushing these individuals to strive for achievement and recognition. Success becomes more than just a goal—it serves as a way to prove their worth, conquer insecurities, or gain approval from others. This determination fuels their ambition and resilience in overcoming setbacks to excel. However, while success can offer temporary validation, the underlying emotional wounds often persist beneath the surface. Understanding this dynamic is crucial in comprehending the complex motivations and journeys of successful individuals, underscoring the importance of personal growth and healing alongside external achievements.

The idea that many successful people are driven by a need to compensate for past wounds or challenges is grounded in psychological theory and research. While no single scientific study definitively proves this theory across all successful individuals, various psychological principles and studies provide insights into related concepts: Achievement Motivation Theory, introduced by psychologist David McClelland, highlights how individuals are driven by core needs such as achievement, affiliation, and power. McClelland's theory suggests that some people pursue success as a result of a deep-seated desire for achievement, often shaped by their early life experiences. This internal drive can profoundly influence their motivation and approach to achieving goals, underscoring the impact of past experiences on present behaviors.

Attachment Theory, pioneered by John Bowlby, examines the long-term effects of early relationships with caregivers on individuals' behaviors and relationships throughout their lives. According to this theory, individuals with insecure attachment styles—such as anxious or avoidant attachments—may seek validation and security through external achievements or relationships. For these individuals, success in their careers or personal endeavors may serve as a means to compensate for feelings of insecurity or inadequacy stemming from early attachment experiences. Bowlby's theory thus illuminates how early relational dynamics can shape later motivations and behaviors in pursuit of emotional security and validation.

Have you noticed repetitive patterns in your relationships, work dynamics, or health struggles? These patterns often stem from unresolved emotions and energetic imbalances rooted in early emotional experiences. By understanding and addressing these subconscious blocks, you can begin to break free from these patterns and move toward a life of greater clarity and empowerment.

Understanding and addressing subconscious blocks is the first step toward unlocking your full potential. As you continue through this book, you will learn practical techniques to identify and clear these blocks, paving the way for personal and spiritual growth. Embrace this journey with an open heart, knowing that each step brings you closer to your true self and the life you are meant to live.

3

Authentic Power

"Authentic power is building something inside of you that is indestructible." — *Anonymous*

What does power mean to you? How comfortable are you with your authentic power? When you think about being powerful, do you feel excited, scared, or uncertain? Do you believe it's possible to be powerful without being controlling or aggressive? How often do you feel truly empowered in your daily life? These questions invite you to reflect deeply on your relationship with power and your sense of self. As soon as we say the word 'power,' many think of 'power over.' Understanding your authentic power is essential for personal growth and spiritual development.

In the journey of personal growth and spiritual development, one of the most profound realizations is understanding that true power and purpose come from recognizing that it's not about you. This concept can be transformative, freeing you from the pressures of ego and aligning you with a higher purpose. When you understand that your actions, decisions, and life path are part of something greater—<u>whether you call it God, the Universe, Source, Spirit, Creator or a Higher Consciousness—you begin to see yourself as a conduit for divine energy and purpose. This is the essence of authentic power.</u>

Throughout this book, I will use the term "the Universe" to refer to God, Source, Spirit, Creator, or Higher Consciousness. My intention is to be inclusive and respectful of all perspectives on a higher power.

Power is a complex concept that has evolved over time, shaped by cultural, social, and gender dynamics. In my work with women, I have observed a recurring phenomenon: 95% of the women I do chakra readings on have a black spot at the bottom back of their solar plexus chakra. (See Chapter 6 for chakra reading description) This spot is linked to generational conditioning that teaches, "It's not okay to be too powerful," "It's not okay to be more powerful than men," or, "It's not okay to be seen as powerful." These deep-seated, subconscious beliefs have been passed down through generations, influencing women's relationship with their own power and preventing them from embracing their authentic power. I have experienced all of these to varying degrees, healing them at deeper layers over the years.

I was surprised, though not entirely, when I touched upon a deeper layer of "it's not okay to be seen as powerful" while writing this book. Who am I to write this book on authentic power? I see now that this has actually been a life's work. I have come from a place of often feeling powerless in many areas of my life to now experiencing myself as a powerful healer, listener, energy mover, grandmother, and spiritual coach.

Where are you at with these beliefs? I invite you to meditate on what you believe about your own power, both consciously and subconsciously. Go even deeper and ask yourself what other emotions or beliefs accompany these thoughts. Any subconscious blocks that exist within the depths of your right brain will hinder your progress in life unless they are released.

It was fairly common in my generation to be taught to not say anything positive about yourself. You wouldn't want to appear boastful or conceited. I remember when I was 40 years old, I was telling my father about an award I received at work. I was the only woman among many men qualified to receive this award, and I won it. I was proud of myself. I accomplished something of value. I told both my parents over the phone, and my father's response was "you're conceited." It was like a knife in my heart. And, it was his own generational conditioning speaking. It had nothing to do with me or my power.

What is your story around authentic power? What were and are the dynamics in your family, at work, or with friends? I am holding the vision for you that you heal any and all unhealthy dynamics and beliefs around your personal power or the power of the Universe moving through you with the methods in this book. This is where the real magic happens.

"You are the Universe, expressing itself as a human for a little while."

— *Eckhart Tolle*

Historically, power dynamics have favored men. For centuries, patriarchal systems dominated societies, with power being equated with dominance, control, and authority—traits traditionally associated with masculinity. Men were often the decision-makers, warriors, and leaders, while women were relegated to supportive and nurturing roles. This historical imbalance created a belief system where female power was suppressed and undervalued, leading to the generational conditioning many women experience today. However, the concept of power is not one-dimensional and should not be confined to traditional masculine traits. Authentic power, especially feminine power, is fundamentally different.

Feminine, or divine feminine power is rooted in qualities such as empathy, intuition, collaboration, and emotional intelligence. It is the ability to nurture, heal, and create, drawing strength from connection rather than control. This form of power values relationships and community, seeing power as something to be shared and amplified through collective effort. It embraces vulnerability as a source of strength and fosters environments where others can thrive. Female power is inherently inclusive and holistic, integrating mind, body, and spirit to bring about profound and sustainable change. By reclaiming and embracing these aspects of power, women can break free from limiting societal norms and step into their true, authentic selves, leading with compassion, wisdom, and resilience.

Whenever I conduct Azarias Group Energy Healing sessions on the topic of power, the women attending often express a desire to feel more powerful, using words like strength, confidence, or leadership in their intentions. They are clear, however, that they do not seek the type of power associated with "power over" others. Once we have accessed and cleared their blocks to authentic power, they are usually amazed at how peaceful and calm true power feels. For them, it is much more about a quiet, inner knowing than an outward expression. While it has the potential to be expressed outwardly, that is not its core nature. When called forth, it can and will be expressed with confidence. Unlike the often aggressive and outward-focused nature of masculine power, authentic feminine power is more introspective, nurturing, and inclusive. It is about creating harmony, fostering growth, and connecting deeply with oneself and others.

The ego often wants to take credit for achievements and feels the weight of failures. It thrives on validation, control, and personal gain. However, living solely from the ego can lead to a life filled with stress, anxiety, and a constant feeling of inadequacy. The shift comes when you realize that your true purpose is not about personal accolades but about allowing a higher power to work through you. This is where authentic power lies—not in the ego, but in being a vessel for something greater. To me, this is the absolute most fulfilling kind of power. It holds no bounds. While

I certainly am not evolved enough to live in this place all the time, I am eternally grateful whenever I experience it, which is always when I am practicing Azarias Energy Healing and other times like spending time in nature, leading meditations, in meditation myself, or, at times while loving and receiving love with others.

One of the biggest challenges is letting go of control. We are conditioned to believe that we must control every aspect of our lives to succeed. However, surrendering to divine power doesn't mean giving up; it means trusting that there is a greater plan at work. This trust allows you to flow with life's events, seeing them as opportunities for growth and service rather than obstacles to overcome. When you see yourself as a conduit for divine energy, your perspective shifts. This type of power is not gender specific. You start to view your talents, skills, and passions as gifts meant to serve a greater purpose. This mindset can transform how you approach your work, relationships, and personal goals. Instead of asking, "What can I get from this?" you begin to ask, "How can I serve? How can I contribute to the greater good?" This shift from ego-driven goals to a purpose-driven life is the hallmark of authentic power.

To align with your higher purpose, it's essential to cultivate practices that connect you with this greater power. Meditation, prayer, energy work, journaling, and spending time in nature can help you tune into the divine guidance that is always available. Listening to your intuition and following the nudges from the Universe can lead you to paths you may not have considered but are aligned with your highest good. A common fear is that if it's not about you, then you don't matter. On the contrary, recognizing that it's not about you magnifies your significance. You become part of a grander design, contributing to a collective purpose that transcends individual accomplishments. Your actions, no matter how small, are integral to the tapestry of the Universe.

Regularly acknowledging the blessings and opportunities that come your way can shift your focus from what you lack to the abundance that surrounds you. Serving your authentic self and others, whether through your work, volunteer activities, or simple acts of kindness, reinforces the idea that you are part of something bigger. Trusting the process means believing that every experience, whether good or bad, is a stepping stone on your journey. Focusing on the effort and intention behind your actions rather than the outcome allows the Universe to guide you to your highest good.

In order for women to tap into their true power, they must clear the blocks that are getting in the way. In my experience, just doing mindset work around being a powerful woman eventually leads to problems because it is only at the level of the mind and often doesn't leave room for natural emotions of fear, sadness, and even hatred to move through us. Clearing deep subconscious blocks is essential to accessing and embodying true feminine power. When these blocks are removed, women can embrace their power in a way that is both peaceful and impactful.

Understanding that it's not about you but about the Universe moving through you is a powerful shift in consciousness. It liberates you from the constraints of the ego and aligns you with a higher purpose. By embracing this mindset, or better still, heartset, you open yourself to endless possibilities, greater fulfillment, and a deeper connection with the divine. Your life becomes a testament to the power of letting go and allowing the Universe to work through you, bringing forth your true potential and purpose. This is the essence of authentic power.

4

Embracing Discovery and Change

"It is not the strongest of the species that survive, nor the most intelligent, but the one most responsive to change."

— Charles Darwin

Perhaps you've picked up this book because you feel a strong urge to shift or make changes in your career or life. Maybe retirement has left you seeking more meaning, or, like I did years ago and discuss in later chapters, you've explored different paths but still feel unfulfilled, find yourself longing for something greater or a general dissatisfaction in life in general. If so, you're in the right place.

Ask yourself: Do you believe you're destined for something more? Has your current career, business, or lifestyle lost its meaning? Has your passion faded? You might find yourself going through the motions at work or in life, feeling unfulfilled or even lost. Yet, deep down, you know you can achieve something great and are meant for something significant. But finding clarity is challenging. Despite journaling, meditating, therapy, or reflecting, answers seem out of reach. You've looked into new careers or education options, but nothing feels quite right. Most frustratingly, you're very aware of some blocks, while others remain hidden in your subconscious, blocking the clarity you seek.

You're not alone in these feelings. Many of us switch careers or make significant life changes multiple times. The story I've shared here is just one critical moment in my journey, leading to even more profound changes. It's about opening yourself up to more, to your greatness and living from a place of purpose, even when the path forward seems unclear.

Subconscious blocks are a natural part of life, emerging when we're ready to confront them. They present opportunities for healing and growth, and this book will guide you through this transformative journey. Within these pages, you'll delve into the science behind subconscious blocks and explore your subconscious to uncover their roots. Understanding where they come from is the first step toward freeing yourself. I'll guide you through spiritual techniques honed over years of practice, helping you navigate and overcome these blocks to achieve personal growth and empowerment.

As you embark on this journey of healing, you'll discover that your blocks hold the keys to unlocking your true potential. Through practice and introspection, you'll learn to transform these obstacles into opportunities for personal growth. Each exercise is crafted to help you uncover hidden talents and strengths. Whether you're an artist, engineer, retiree, coach, surfer, grandmother, or healer, your purpose contributes to shaping our world.

Keep reading, engage with the exercises, and begin this transformative journey. By addressing your subconscious blocks, you'll unlock your potential and step into a future brimming with possibilities. Embrace this journey, as it reveals your true and authentic self along with your divine purpose.

This book is an invitation for those dedicated to personal and spiritual growth. It's designed for individuals ready to embrace authentic spiritual work, even when it challenges their beliefs about themselves and the world. Within these pages, you will discover how to access and understand your subconscious, uncovering hidden blocks, wounds, and traumas. Clearing away this stagnant energy is crucial to allowing your true self to shine. This book encourages you to live consciously and purposefully.

Are you ready to delve into your subconscious, using hidden blocks and wounds as stepping stones? Immerse yourself in these pages and empower yourself to live your soul's purpose in extraordinary ways. You sense something is holding you back. Perhaps you've identified some blocks, but the most significant ones—those stifling your potential—are still hidden. You know you're meant for more and yearn for the fulfillment that comes with realizing your potential. But clarity remains elusive. Despite glimpses of your path, the full picture stays just out of reach.

Like many, you've attended workshops, therapy sessions, or hired coaches, hoping for a breakthrough, yet you're still frustrated and grappling with unseen barriers. You know you have more to offer, but overcoming these blocks feels overwhelming. By selecting this book, you're demonstrating your dedication to change and growth. Congratulations on this commitment; let's delve deeper.

This book serves as a guiding light through uncertainty, designed for those who sense there's more to life but aren't sure how to reach it. Within these pages, embark on a transformative journey, uncovering subconscious blocks and finding clarity and fulfillment.

Over my 30-year journey, I've developed spiritual practices for healing and empowerment through meditation and self-healing. This book is for those ready for change and committed to deep internal work.

You may already be familiar with chakras—energy centers in your body that help regulate physical, emotional, and spiritual well-being. There are seven main chakras, each located at a specific point along the inside of your spine and associated with different functions.

Like many, I first meditated on the chakras in front of my body. Initially, this practice was enlightening and brought me a sense of peace and balance. However, as I delved deeper into my meditation practice, I began to seek more profound experiences and deeper connections within my body.

One day, during a particularly introspective meditation session, I decided to shift my focus. Instead of visualizing the chakras at the front of my body, I brought my awareness inside my body, specifically to the center of my body, in front of my spine. To my surprise, this simple change amplified my experiences significantly. The sensations were more intense, the energy flow more vibrant, and the sense of healing and empowerment within myself more profound.

As I continued this practice, I noticed remarkable changes not only in my meditation sessions but also in my daily life. The heightened awareness and intensified energy flow seemed to resonate throughout my entire being, bringing about a deeper sense of healing and clarity.

Later, as I began performing energy healings on others, I observed a similar pattern. Initially, when guiding my clients to breathe into their chakras, they would naturally focus on the front of their bodies, just as I had initially done. The results were beneficial, but I sensed there was more potential to unlock. So, I began instructing them to shift their focus to the chakras within the inside of the spine.

The results were nothing short of extraordinary. Clients reported more profound healing experiences, deeper emotional releases, and a heightened sense of joy, hope, freedom, authentic power, etc. It was as if tuning into the core of their chakras allowed them to access a more potent and transformative energy.

Inspired by these outcomes, I fully embraced this approach in my own meditation practice. I now meditate on the chakras along the inside of the spine, believing this to be the true center of each chakra. Except for the third eye, which I focus on in the center of the head, this method has become my standard practice and what I teach.

These chakras are always open. We cannot close them, just like we cannot shut down any of our organs. What we can do is focus on them and activate their energy to a higher level. It is kind of like massaging one of your organs or taking a supplement to help it function better. I have been doing chakra readings for years and most people are blown away by the amount of information they are provided with about themselves and their lives. In this book, explore how to work with chakras for healing and transformation.

I encourage you to try this approach as well. By focusing on the chakras along the spine, you can amplify your experiences and unlock deeper levels of healing and transformation. It's a subtle shift that can bring about significant changes, offering you the most profound benefits from your meditation practice. Give it a try, and you might find that this inward focus provides the best bang for your buck.

Understanding the precise location of each chakra can further enhance your practice. Let's explore the specific positions of the chakras to deepen your connection and maximize your meditation's effectiveness.

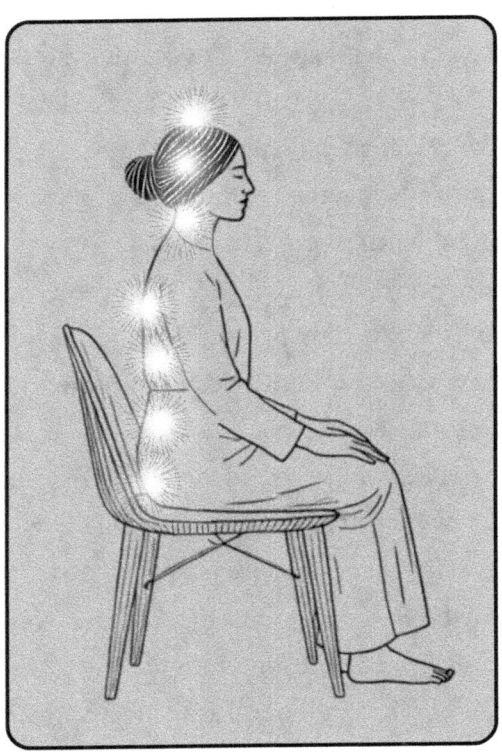

Chakra Locations:

- **Root Chakra:** Located at the base of your spine, and to me, it's about firstly, safety and stability, which, when well developed, moves into trust and faith and when this is well developed, moves into responsibility and accomplishment. The highest level of this being what your soul chose to be responsible for accomplishing in this lifetime.
- **Sacral Chakra:** Found a couple of inches below your navel, this chakra deals with creativity, intimacy, passion, and one-on-one relationships, especially with the mother.
- **Solar Plexus Chakra:** Located in your upper stomach area, just below the sternum, it's all about truth and power. Truth is power and it is not only personal truth and power, but divine truth and power moving through you. It is also known as the deep heart.
- **Heart Chakra:** Positioned in the center of your chest, it governs love and compassion.
- **Throat Chakra:** Found in your throat, this chakra is about being seen and heard. The highest level is about the expression of your soul's purpose.
- **Third Eye Chakra:** Located between your eyebrows, it deals with intuition and insight.
- **Crown Chakra:** Found at the top of your head, it connects you to higher consciousness and the cosmos.

Are you ready to commit to this journey of discovery and transformation? It requires effort, but the rewards are immense. Your efforts here will enhance your self-awareness and resilience, guiding you through life's challenges. What is your intention? What would you like to gain from reading and doing the practices in this book?

Take some time now to reflect on this, meditate, or journal. It will help you clarify your goals and set a powerful intention for your journey. Write down your thoughts and feelings about what you hope to achieve. This reflection will serve as a guide and a source of motivation as you progress. Here is a brief meditation to assist you:

Meditation for Setting Your Intention

Find a quiet space where you can sit comfortably and won't be disturbed. Close your eyes and take a few deep breaths, allowing your body to relax with each exhale. Begin to focus on your breath. Inhale deeply through your nose, feeling your abdomen rise. Exhale slowly through your nose, feeling your body release any tension. As you continue to breathe deeply, bring to mind your intention for this journey. Tune into all the emotions you feel around feeling blocked or the reason(s) you are reading this book. Acknowledge everything, especially those difficult emotions that are at the core of where you are at today.

Then, I invite you to imagine you have finished reading this book and have completed all the practices. What emotions are you experiencing knowing you have cleared many subconscious blocks and you have stepped into a much more authentically powerful version of yourself?

Connect with these emotions and notice if there are any deeper, positive emotions. Let these positive emotions be your goal. Whether it is joy, peace, empowerment, unconditional love or success, let these feelings fill your entire being. Silently or aloud, repeat an affirmation that resonates with your emotional intention. It could be something like, "My intention is to feel vibrant, unstoppable, beautiful and powerful or ?

Silently or aloud, repeat an affirmation that resonates with your emotional intention. This affirmation could be something like, "I am vibrant, unstoppable, beautiful, and powerful." Alternatively, you might choose a different affirmation that feels right for you, such as, "I am grounded in my purpose, radiant with inner peace, and overflowing with limitless potential."

By using a variety of affirmations, you open yourself to a broader range of positive experiences and emotions. Allow yourself to experiment and find the affirmation that most deeply resonates with your current state of being. Embrace these affirmations as a way to cultivate and reinforce the powerful, authentic version of yourself that you are becoming.

And how committed are you to yourself and your process regardless of the challenges. Here's an example: "I am open to growth and transformation," or "I am committed to discovering my true self and living authentically."

After spending a few minutes in this visualization and affirmation, gently release your intention to the Universe. Trust that your journey will unfold as it should, and that you are supported every step of the way. Slowly bring your awareness back to the present moment. Wiggle your fingers and toes, and when you're ready, open your eyes. Take a moment to sit quietly and reflect on your experience.

Write down any insights, feelings, or thoughts that came up during your meditation. This will help you solidify your intention and provide a reference point as you progress through the book.

By clearly understanding your intentions, you'll be better equipped to focus on the practices and exercises that resonate most deeply with you. This clarity will empower you to embrace the journey with an open heart and a willing spirit, uncovering the clarity and purpose you've been seeking. Your transformation starts right here, right now. Embrace this journey with courage and determination, and you'll discover the incredible potential within you.

I am here with you and I've designed this process to be as safe and supportive as possible, ensuring that you feel empowered to embrace the fullness of who you are. Together, we'll unlock the potential within you and set it into motion, transforming your aspirations into tangible actions.

You have just taken the first step toward a more empowered, fulfilling life. Your journey of transformation is now in flow. I invite you to embrace the journey with an open heart and a willing spirit, and together we'll uncover the clarity and purpose you've been seeking.

5

How I Cleared My Blocks, Gained Clarity & Started Living My Purpose (the first time)

"The first step towards getting somewhere is to decide you're not going to stay where you are." — J.P. Morgan

Almost 30 years ago, I had just been recognized as the top salesperson for the BC Power Smart Home Improvement Program in my region. The excitement from the award quickly faded, and the next day, like most days, I felt an intense longing for something more meaningful. What had once been a role full of valuable learning and growth—helping others improve their homes' energy efficiency and air quality—no longer fulfilled me like it once had. For nine years, I had worked in this job, earning enough to support my two children and myself without child support from my ex. I set my own hours, we enjoyed wonderful vacations, occasionally went out for dinner, and outwardly, it seemed like I had everything together as a single mother.

Inside, however, I felt like I was slowly withering. The work that used to be fulfilling and somewhat exciting no longer sparked much joy in me. To counter this, I tried different activities: stained glass, new types of yoga, joined groups, and went on more kayaking trips. I regularly led a meditation group, where I facilitated sessions to deepen inner peace, and practiced shamanic techniques for my spiritual growth and to help others heal. Although these activities were enjoyable, they didn't ease my dissatisfaction with my day job. I felt lost. Even though I searched for other work, nothing resonated or offered enough pay. I realized I was meant for more than my current job provided, but I had no idea what that "more" could be. I was completely blocked from imagining any new or exciting possibilities. While it was rewarding to help transform unhealthy homes on Vancouver Island into healthier environments by addressing mold, ventilation issues, and poor insulation, it no longer brought the same sense of fulfillment.

For about eight months, another company had been trying to recruit me. Feeling unappreciated at my current job, I decided to switch. I didn't regret it. I got my own office—a beautiful space with glass walls on two sides. My opinions on products were valued, and I felt appreciated. The general manager encouraged me to co-host a Saturday morning radio show with him. Although I initially declined, I eventually agreed and had a lot of fun doing it with him. I started to feel fulfilled again, but this feeling was short-lived. Something was still missing; I continued to long for something more, something that would align with my soul's true purpose.

I vividly remember a Tuesday after the August long weekend when I returned to work and found a new general manager in the office. To this day, I have never seen anyone with such cold eyes. I distinctly remember thinking, "This man has shark eyes." The previous general manager had been demoted to sales manager, and the new general manager took charge. He soon called me into his office to discuss changes, including switching to lower-grade products while maintaining the same prices to boost revenue. I knew immediately that I could not support this. I had to believe in the products I was offering to my clients. Fear welled up inside me. I went to my office and meditated. I knew I would be out of personal integrity if I stayed. I gave notice, despite not having any idea what I would do next. Nervous but resolute, I informed him that I was giving three to four weeks' notice to allow time for my replacement. His response was blunt: "No, you can leave right now." When I expressed concern about my ongoing projects, he simply said, "Don't worry about it; it will all be taken care of." I packed up my office and left. I drove to the forest near my home which I visited almost daily. It was my spiritual temple. I cried my eyes out, then picked myself up and thought, somehow, this is going to be a new beginning. A few months later, the owner of the company arranged a lunch meeting, almost pleading for my return after experiencing a considerable drop in sales. He even produced a large check with my name on it to entice me. I agreed to rejoin, but only if "Mr. Shark Eyes," was let go. My conditional offer was declined.

It was summer vacation for my children. I told them what had happened and announced that we were going camping, and they could each bring a friend. I knew this would give me the space to think and plan my next steps. We had a wonderful time at the ocean, boogie boarding, sitting around the campfire, picking fresh blackberries every day, and exploring more of Vancouver Island.

During this time, I meditated, sought guidance, and journaled my thoughts. Although I came up with some ideas, none felt right. Back home, I continued exploring other job opportunities, but nothing clicked.

Something had to change. I couldn't stay unemployed much longer. I decided I needed to go on a deeper journey of self-discovery. I dedicated myself to an even longer morning meditation practice, spent time journaling, and opened myself up with surrender to find a more fulfilling career path. I knew I had blocks to discovering or creating what was next for me, but I had no idea what they were. Each morning, I set aside time for meditation, allowing myself to sink into a state of deep introspection and connection with my inner guidance. Through this practice, I developed and refined over time a process which is now shared in this book. I cleared some blocks, something I had been practicing successfully for some time, but not with respect to my career or purpose in life. I also slowly cultivated a sense of clarity and insight, gradually unraveling the layers of my being to uncover my true desires and aspirations. Finally, I embraced the concept of surrender, letting go of my attachment to preconceived notions of what was available to me, and allowing the Universe to guide me toward my true calling. In this state of openness and receptivity, I found the courage to stay open to discovering and pursuing a career aligned with my authentic self, paving the way for a journey of fulfillment and purpose. I still didn't know what that would be, but I was so much more open and hopeful. I felt I was closer to stepping into my greatness and living my soul's true purpose.

One day, as I was leaving a store, I noticed a community college calendar in a stand. My intuition urged me to pick it up, but I initially dismissed the idea, thinking, "I have two kids; I can't go back to school." I walked out of the store. Once outside, I could still feel the pull of the calendar. It was so strong that I turned around, went back in, grabbed it, and put it in my bag. Once home, I made myself a cup of tea and opened the calendar to their interior design program. "What?" I thought. I had no idea such a program was available so close to home. As I read about it, I realized I was very qualified. There was an open house scheduled for the following week. I questioned how I could possibly return to school, given my responsibilities.

As a single mother, I often spent weekends painting, sewing, renovating, and decorating my house. I grew up with parents who were always decorating and renovating. This had been part of my life every year up until. I loved interior design and everything associated with it. Despite initial hesitations, I attended the open house, deciding it was worth seeing what they had to say. Listening to the instructors, I felt compelled to find a way to enroll. I went to the bank and was astonished to learn they would loan me the money for tuition, and even enough to make the loan payments! My savings would cover the rest of my expenses. Realizing I couldn't say no, I was overwhelmed with joy and eagerly awaited the start of classes. I completed the program with an award for overall excellence and successfully ran my own business for a decade. In a marketing class, when I declared my target market as spiritual women, the instructor cautioned that I might only attract 20% of potential clients. My response? "Well, that's the 20% I want to work with." Truthfully, not all my clients were spiritual, but those who embraced spirituality were such a joy to work with.

Through my business, "Stelte Design: Designing for the Soul", I integrated spirituality with interior design and decorating. My mission was to help people reflect their true selves in their environments, their homes, and personal spaces. My goal was to help them discover clarity about who they truly were. I also engaged in a lot of spiritual work, which I will share more about later. Reflecting on my journey, I wish I had this book earlier in my career. Stelte Design was my first big career shift. It was the one that prepared me to discover, embrace, and live my true life purpose. Here's the rest of the story.

My business thrived on referrals, and I wholeheartedly embraced each client and their wishes. One notable referral came from a client who sought a complete home makeover after her husband's passing. Our collaboration involved significant spiritual exploration, leading her on a journey of self-discovery. She referred me to a friend in Vancouver, and despite the considerable travel involved, I accepted the invitation. I'll call her Chris. Chris presented as a confident, professional woman who had it all together. She proceeded to take me around her home and told me all the things she was unhappy with. She and her husband had been remodeling this house for a few years, and they were at their wit's end. She couldn't seem to make any decisions around the finishing touches, with furniture or its placement, window treatments, art, and was struggling with what to get rid of and what to keep. I was surprised at how indecisive she was. As she went on, she just seemed lost. She asked me if it would be best if they just sold the house.

I gave her all the design advice I could, which she appreciated. Even with some decisions made, she still seemed confused. I asked her if she would like me to do a spiritual reading for her, to gain insight and clarity around her home. She remembered that her friend who referred her did some spiritual work with me and she decided she would appreciate the reading. Time had passed and I had to get back on the ferry to go home, so we agreed that I would do the reading back in Victoria and then follow up on Monday with the results. Back then I would do readings for my clients on the beach sitting on a log. Being at the ocean seemed to help with receptivity. I did receive some helpful guidance around the antique dining room table that she wanted to keep and what I kept being shown was a bouquet of white chrysanthemums in a beautiful vase on the table. I knew it was significant because I was shown the same image multiple times. When we spoke on Monday, she seemed to appreciate everything I shared with her, but went silent every time I mentioned the white chrysanthemums. Finally, I asked her if the white chrysanthemums meant anything to her. She started to cry. She told me that her wedding bouquet was all white chrysanthemums and that she and her husband had been talking about divorce. I get goosebumps, as always, when I remember her saying. "This tells me that we are meant to stay together, that our relationship is much more important than the house. I am so grateful for this."

They stayed together. She was able to put her attention on her marriage and let go of her need for the house and its belongings being perfect. I continued to help her with the finishing details on their home, helping her discover more of her true self and express that in her home. When I visited her later, I asked her if she was still considering selling her house. She looked surprised and said, "No, I've never thought about it since our first meeting." The result was a space that was not only beautiful but a reflection of her truest self. I realized the power of combining my skills with my spiritual gifts, leading to a profound sense of fulfillment.

Looking back, it was the combination of healing my wounds which cleared my blocks to discover my true self and access more and more of my authentic power that led me to discover my soul's purpose here on earth. The journey was not easy, and there were moments of uncertainty and fear, but each step brought me closer to living a life of purpose and fulfillment.

I'm here to support you on your journey of transformation, to help you clear the blocks that are holding you back, and to empower you to step into your greatness. You can trust that your soul's purpose is waiting to be discovered, and you will have the strength within you to embrace it fully.

As you complete this chapter, remember that mastering the Full Breath is the first step in becoming your own energy worker. This powerful practice not only calms your mind and body but also serves as a gateway to your subconscious, where true healing and transformation begin. By committing to the Full Breath, you are laying the groundwork for profound personal growth, allowing you to clear old patterns, access your inner wisdom, and step into your authentic power. Embrace this journey with dedication, and you will discover the limitless potential within you to create the life you desire.

6

First Step to Becoming Your Own Energy Worker

"When you learn how to harness the power of your energy, you can create the life you want."

— *Anonymous*

Throughout this book, we will be using the Full Breath in every meditation. Before diving into why it's crucial to breathe fully during meditation, I want to share how I first discovered the Full Breath.

Growing up in Edmonton, Alberta, Canada, the winters were bitterly cold, and it was common to have three feet or more of snow on the ground for months. When I was about eight years old, I was walking to a friend's house one winter day. The cold was so intense that I started shivering uncontrollably. To warm up, I began walking faster, which made my breath quicken, and soon I was panting, switching from nose breathing to mouth breathing.

I remembered my mom often telling us never to breathe through our mouths in the cold because it could freeze our lungs. I had my scarf wrapped tightly around my face, covering everything but my eyes. I was caught between trying not to freeze my lungs and not wanting my body to get any colder. In my struggle to maintain a fast pace while breathing through my nose, I discovered that taking longer breaths through my nose allowed me to walk quickly and stopped my shivering. To my surprise, this slower, deeper breathing also made me feel a bit warmer as my body relaxed.

Whenever I started to pant and breathe more quickly, the shivering would return, and I would feel colder. This simple yet profound discovery made a huge difference, and I began using that breath every winter from then on.

Later, in junior high, I used the same long, steady nose breathing while running laps around the track. It helped me build better endurance, and I even taught it to a few classmates who found it helpful too.

Incorporating this breathing style into my meditation practice became second nature. I didn't fully understand all its benefits back then, but I knew it felt right, even when my instructors said it wasn't necessary. That was over 30 years ago, and the Full Breath has been a foundational part of my practice ever since.

Long, full belly breaths are not just calming—they are powerful tools for accessing the subconscious mind. This is not just spiritual wisdom but is also supported by neuroscience and psychology. Understanding how deep breathing affects brain function and emotional regulation can illuminate why it is a key practice in accessing and clearing subconscious blocks.

Breathing with the lower abdomen with long, Full Breaths significantly impacts brain function by shifting the control of breathing from the medulla oblongata to the frontal lobe. The medulla oblongata, located in the brainstem, is responsible for involuntary functions, including automatic breathing. However, when we consciously engage in deep abdominal breathing, the frontal lobe, which is involved in higher-order thinking, decision-making, and self-awareness, begins to take over the regulation of breath.

By actively using the abdominal muscles, we move from automatic, shallow breathing controlled by the medulla oblongata to more deliberate and mindful breathing controlled by the frontal lobe. This conscious control activates the vagus nerve and enhances our ability to focus and remain present, freeing up the medulla oblongata from its default task of managing breath. As a result, the brainstem can facilitate access to deeper brain functions, including the subconscious mind.

When the medulla oblongata is relieved of its primary role in breathing regulation, it allows for better autonomic balance and a more profound state of relaxation. This shift promotes the brain's alpha and theta wave activity, which are associated with states of deep relaxation, meditation, and increased creativity. These brain wave patterns are crucial for accessing the subconscious mind, where deep-seated memories, emotions, wounds, traumas, and beliefs reside.

In essence, breathing with the lower abdomen initiates a neurophysiological shift that enhances cognitive control, promotes relaxation, and facilitates access to the subconscious. This practice not only helps reduce stress and anxiety but also provides a powerful tool for self-exploration and healing, allowing individuals to uncover and transform subconscious patterns that influence their thoughts and behaviors. Through this process, we can tap into our inner wisdom and promote profound personal growth and transformation.

The Full Breath is more than a technique; it's a practice of engaging the entire breath cycle with intention and awareness to access the deeper layers of the self. We always begin by sitting comfortably on a chair, like a kitchen or dining chair. You will need to ensure your back is straight and your head is held high with your chin level. This posture creates a direct, unobstructed path for energy to flow along your spine. Why does that matter?

<u>What I notice in people when I do chakra readings is that the bulk of their wounding and trauma is energetically held along the inside of the spine or around it. This area is a central conduit for both physical and energetic communication within the body.</u>

<u>The spine houses various energetic pathways that run up and down the spine.</u>

The flow of vital energy and the conduits in our bodies containing and guiding this flow have been studied for centuries. In yogic and tantric traditions, the shushumna, ida, and pingala nadis are seen as essential components of the subtle energy system. The nadis originate from the base of the spine and are closely associated with the chakras and the flow of prana (life force energy) throughout the body. The shushumna nadi is the central channel that runs along the spinal column from the base of the spine (the root chakra) to the crown of the head (the crown chakra). It is considered the primary channel for the flow of spiritual energy.

The ida nadi starts at the base of the spine, at the root chakra, and winds its way up the left side of the spine, crossing the shushumna nadi at each chakra. It is associated with lunar energy, representing calmness, cooling, and feminine qualities. Ida energy is often connected with the left nostril and the right hemisphere of the brain. The pingala nadi also originates at the base of the spine, at the root chakra, and ascends the right side of the spine, intersecting the shushumna nadi at each chakra. It is associated with solar energy, representing activity, heating, and masculine qualities. Pingala is often connected with the right nostril and the left hemisphere of the brain.

These three nadis are crucial for balancing the body's energy system, and practices like pranayama (breathing exercises), meditation, and yoga aim to harmonize their flow to achieve physical, mental, and spiritual well-being.

Energetically, the spine serves as the main support structure for our body's alignment, not just physically but emotionally and spiritually as well. Trauma and wounding often manifest as blockages or imbalances within the chakras, which are the energy centers distributed along the spine from the base to the crown. These blockages can impede the natural flow of energy, leading to various physical, emotional, and mental health issues.

In Traditional Chinese Medicine, the meridians are similar to the nadis in that they are energy channels. The bladder meridian, which runs along the sides of the spine, is closely associated with stored fear and stress. This meridian plays a crucial role in the body's ability to process and release these emotions. When there is an energetic blockage or imbalance in the spine, it can affect the entire meridian system, amplifying feelings of fear and anxiety. My acupressure teacher used to call it the "meridian of fear," as it is where our unresolved issues tend to accumulate when we "put our problems behind us."

I mentioned earlier that I do chakra readings. So what is a chakra reading? Imagine gaining a deeper understanding of your energy flow and uncovering the hidden blocks that may be holding you back. A chakra reading can illuminate your path, revealing your strengths and guiding you towards greater fulfillment, authenticity, and clarity. By signing up for a chakra reading, you take a proactive step towards personal growth and healing, empowering yourself to live a more vibrant and fulfilled life.

The way I see energy in the chakras is as light (bright light) and dark (black or gray). Seeing the chakras is a skill I developed over time, not a skill I was born with and I teach this technique to others. Kirlian photography has shown that we are beings of light, confirming our nature as energetic beings. The light represents areas where energy is flowing well, often highlighting our superpowers. The black or gray indicates where our blocks are. I view the chakras from multiple perspectives, each symbolic: the top, bottom, sides, front, back, and middle. Using my intuition, I access the meanings of where the energy flows freely and where it is stuck. I also delve into why it is flowing the way it is or why it is blocked, providing insights into what you can do about it.

Chakra readings are something I always love to do because they provide much-needed clarity. Most of us seek understanding around our blocks and how we might improve or move forward in work, relationships, health, or life in general. If you are looking for clarity, you have come to the right place.

Problems a Chakra Reading Can Solve

Identifying Energetic Blocks: Pinpoint areas where your energy is stuck, which may be affecting your emotional, mental or physical well-being.

Enhancing Self-Awareness: Gain a deeper understanding of your inner strengths and potential, often referred to as your "superpowers."

Improving Life Areas: Receive guidance on how to move forward in specific areas of your life, such as career, relationships, or personal growth.

My goal is to let you know where the energetic blocks are and where the energy is flowing well. I am often able to see what your superpowers are. I will give you some ideas around how to help yourself with your energy flow in the chakras and more.

If that feels right, here's a QR code for you to use to sign up for a chakra reading. If now is not the time, a reading will be available if or when you want it. Or, here is the link:

https://cherylstelte.kartra.com/calendar/25chakra

The next step is for you to practice the Full Breath.

Full Breath Meditation

Start by placing one hand on your lower abdomen, with your thumb resting at your navel. This hand placement serves as a guide to help you focus on breathing deeply into your lower abdomen. As you inhale slowly through your nose, count to six or eight seconds, allowing your abdomen to expand outward. This movement should be gentle and natural, avoiding any significant rise in your shoulders or much movement in your chest. After reaching the peak of your inhale, immediately begin the exhale without a pause. Exhale slowly through your nose for the same count of six to eight seconds.

Focus on completely expelling the air from your lungs. Try pushing more air out even when you think your exhalation is finished. Most people hold onto this last bit of air and never fully exhale. This full exhalation is crucial because it clears out the carbon dioxide and stale air, creating space for fresh, oxygen-rich air. Incomplete exhalation can lead to shallow breathing, limiting oxygen intake and contributing to a sense of anxiety or tension. By fully releasing each breath, you also let go of physical and emotional stress, and whatever no longer serves you energetically, promoting relaxation and balance.

Embracing this method can unlock your potential and help you tap into the rich reservoir of your subconscious mind. In a relaxed state, the mind's psychological defenses—such as repression and denial—are lowered. This reduced defensiveness allows suppressed memories and emotions to surface more easily, making them available for conscious processing. It creates an internal environment where subconscious material can be accessed and integrated without the usual resistance.

Another great benefit of the Full Breath is that it enhances neuroplasticity, which is essential for reprogramming subconscious patterns. With improved neuroplasticity, the brain is better equipped to form new neural pathways and break free from old patterns of thought and behavior. This makes it possible to replace limiting subconscious beliefs with empowering ones.

Deep breathing enhances oxygenation throughout the body, including the brain. More oxygen-rich blood flowing to the brain improves cognitive functions such as concentration, clarity, and memory. This oxygen boost can also enhance neuroplasticity—the brain's ability to reorganize itself by forming new neural connections, which is essential for processing and integrating new information.

Chronic stress and anxiety can create mental noise that makes it difficult to access the subconscious mind. Belly breathing (another term that describes the Full Breath practice) lowers levels of cortisol, the body's primary stress hormone. Lower cortisol levels reduce anxiety and help clear the mental fog that often accompanies stress.

Belly breathing fosters a strong connection between the mind and body. This practice improves your internal awareness and your ability to perceive internal body states. Enhanced internal awareness helps you become more attuned to subtle physiological and emotional signals, making it easier to recognize and address subconscious blocks.

By mastering the Full Breath, you lay a solid foundation for becoming your own energy worker. This technique will empower you to access deeper layers of your subconscious, facilitating profound personal growth and healing. I recommend starting with a minimum of 10 minutes for the Full Breath and gradually working up to 20 minutes daily. Embrace this practice with intention and dedication, and you will unlock the potential within you to transform your life and step into your authentic power.

7

Accessing and Clearing Subconscious Blocks

"Your task is not to seek for love, but merely to seek and find all the barriers within yourself that you have built against it." — *Rumi*

Accessing and clearing subconscious blocks is a crucial step in your journey towards empowerment and healing. By identifying and addressing the deep-seated obstacles in your subconscious, you can unlock your true potential and achieve greater clarity and purpose.

Testimonial: "I went to Cheryl to get help with sorting out and putting into action the next steps in my spiritual development, and also to work on physical and emotional health issues with a healer who could see energy. Cheryl has been amazing on both counts. She can see and read both the health and damage located in our chakras, and she can then guide her clients through a healing process specific to what she finds. My spiritual growth and physical/emotional health are being supported now in a beautiful way that comes from within my soul, and I have a much deeper understanding of healing trauma and childhood neglect. Cheryl is a gentle and empathic healer who listens well and uses her ability to see energy in a powerful way." —Sherilyn

This testimonial illustrates the effectiveness of the methods discussed in this chapter and provides a personal account of how accessing and clearing subconscious blocks can lead to significant improvements in spiritual growth and physical/emotional health.

In this chapter, we will use the Full Breath to help access and clear subconscious blocks, allowing you to create space in your subconscious for your authentic power to be ignited. When I first started using the Full Breath in my meditations, I didn't fully understand its benefits. However, it wasn't long before the wounds and traumas of my past began to surface, and I learned to clear them.

At the beginning of my meditation journey, I was severely depressed and taking antidepressants. This was in the early 1990s when diagnosing depression was becoming more common and mainstream in western medicine. After about three months of meditating, my intuition suggested that I could stop taking the antidepressants. My doctor advised against it, but I decided to go off them anyway. Since my meditation practice was still new and not yet a daily routine, I noticed that if I stopped meditating for a week, I would start feeling down again. Once I resumed, I felt better.

I realized that meditation was crucial for my well-being and decided to make meditation my medicine. Since then, I have meditated every day. My doctor remained surprised for years afterward, that I was no longer depressed. He often had me fill out questionnaires to assess my mental health, which consistently showed positive results. He would shake his head in amazement and tell me to keep doing what I was doing. I am certainly not suggesting anyone who is taking medications of any kind to go off them and replace with meditation without the supervision of a doctor. I was only on the anti-depressants for a few months before I went off. What I suggest is that if you are taking any medication and want to stop, build up your meditation practice and speak with your doctor.

The Full Breath became an essential part of my healing and self-care, helping me maintain emotional balance and clear the deep-seated blocks that had weighed me down. Through consistent practice, you too can experience the profound benefits of using the Full Breath in meditation to clear subconscious obstacles and enhance your overall well-being.

Now we'll apply the Full Breath technique to access and clear subconscious blocks. This process is essential for gaining clarity because hidden obstacles act as unseen barriers. They prevent us from reaching our full potential, understanding our true desires, and making decisions that align with our highest goals.

To effectively address and clear subconscious blocks, I developed what I call The ACE Method: The Power of Clearing Subconscious Blocks. ACE stands for Access, Clear, and Empower. It will help you overcome the barriers holding you back and provide the clarity you need to move forward. While the concepts presented here are straight forward and may seem familiar, there's a significant difference between merely understanding ideas and actively implementing them. This method emphasizes not just knowing, but doing—taking action, creating, and energetically attracting the change your heart truly desires. This method is accomplished through meditation with the Full Breath.

First, Access involves identifying and becoming aware of your subconscious blocks by paying attention to the emotions and/or physical sensations that arise during the Full Breath. This in turn allows you to access your right, subconscious brain. You can then trace wounds or blocks back to their origins. Accessing the Energetic Blocks in Your Subconscious is not just a preliminary step; it's a fundamental cornerstone for embarking on your journey of self-discovery and personal growth. Recognizing the unprocessed, trapped emotions can pave the way for profound transformation.

Next, Clear means working on releasing these blocks. The goal here is to confront and process the underlying traumas or wounds using the Full Breath. Remember trauma is stored in the right brain through physical sensations, emotions and fragmented memories. You will learn to breathe through these in order to release blocks from your system permanently without having to relive the events fully.

Finally, Empower entails replacing old patterns with new, empowering emotions, beliefs, and behaviors. This is about building a new foundation of trust, safety, and purpose in your life. It enables you to move forward with confidence and clarity. This is how you step into your greatness and live your soul's purpose.

Understanding your subconscious blocks and how they affect your life is crucial for personal growth and healing. By applying the ACE Method, you can begin to clear these barriers and empower yourself, taking the first steps toward a more aligned and fulfilling life. Remember, this journey requires patience and persistence. Be gentle with yourself as you continue to explore and heal.

The ACE Method Meditation is broken up below into three sections so you can learn it in pieces. Once you practice this meditation frequently, it will eventually become automatic for you to naturally go through the steps of Access, Clear and Empower.

> *"The wound is the place where the Light enters you."*
>
> *— Rumi*

A is for ACCESS Meditation:

Begin by taking a moment to reflect on your intention. What are you seeking to achieve through this meditation of self-discovery? Are there recurring challenges or unfulfilled desires in your life that you wish to understand better or overcome? Pose these inquiries to yourself, allowing your inner wisdom to guide you towards a simple intention of what you would like to accomplish through this meditation.

Assume a relaxed yet grounded posture, sitting in a chair with your spine straight and your hands resting gently on your lap. Close your eyes and bring your awareness to your breath, focusing on the rhythmic rise and fall of your lower abdomen. If this practice is new to you, I invite you to place your hand on your lower abdomen with your thumb at the level of your navel, following the instructions for the Full Breath above.

Remember, our usual breathing patterns often keep us anchored in the left side of the brain, where logical thought predominates. However, by engaging the abdominal muscles and practicing deep, intentional breaths, we can shift our brain function to access the right side, where the subconscious mind resides. This shift is crucial, as the subconscious is where unresolved trauma and emotional wounds are stored, recalled not through linear memory but through physical sensations and emotions.

Commit to practicing long, Full Breaths, inhaling deeply for a count of 6-8 seconds, and exhaling slowly for the same duration until this becomes comfortable.

Bring your awareness down to your root chakra. It's ideal to start here because this is the center of safety and stability and accessing and clearing blocks here will help all the chakras above it.

Keep your internal eyes in the chakra while maintaining the Full Breath.

Ask yourself probing questions to yourself during your full-breath meditation, allowing yourself to explore the emotions that may be hindering you at your core:

- *What is it that I don't want to feel?*
- *What is the emotion that is getting in my way?*
- *What emotion did I feel when _____ happened?*
- *What uncomfortable or difficult emotions am I resisting or suppressing?*
- *When did I first experience these emotions?*
- *What physical sensations, if any, do I notice in my body?*
- *Notice any fragmented memories or events that come up and ask what were the emotions?*

Whatever emotions come up for you are true. Try not to question or resist them and instead, sink into them, feeling them completely for a few minutes each. Once you breathe through one emotion, look for another emotion underneath that one. This is what I call "following the emotional thread." Take the time to breathe into each emotion for a few minutes, following the emotional thread until a new emotion doesn't surface.

Next, staying with the last emotion, allow yourself, still using the Full Breath, to drift back in time to when this emotion first began, likely before the age of 10 or even 5. Give yourself all the time you need. Once you arrive at a certain time in your life, still feeling your emotion, imagine becoming that younger self and breathe into the emotion at whatever age you have drifted back to. It doesn't have to be exact and can be approximate, for example - sometime between the age of 4 and 6. Continue to breathe into the emotion as your younger self until the emotion has dissipated. Remember you don't have to remember what happened.

Follow the emotional thread again to see if there are deeper emotions held at this age. Children usually don't process their emotions well on their own, so the emotions stay stuck until they are touched into as an adult.

C - CLEAR

Clearing the Energetic Subconscious Blocks is not only essential but also foundational for your emotional well-being, shaping your experiences from the earliest stages of life. Research has revealed that humans begin experiencing emotions, including those transmitted by their mothers, even while in the womb. Positive emotions trigger the release of oxytocin, nurturing bonding and emotional connection, while stress and trauma can prompt the release of cortisol, potentially impacting emotional development.

From my extensive personal and professional experience, I've witnessed profound healing transformations, with the journey often commencing as early as the prenatal stages. To embark on your own journey of clearing these energetic blocks, I recommend starting with a deep belly breath, an ancient practice with profound effects on emotional release and energetic balance.

To effectively clear subconscious blocks, it's crucial to engage with all emotions and physical sensations in a mindful and accepting manner. Emotions often carry deep messages from our subconscious, and fully experiencing them is key to releasing their hold on our psyche. When you encounter emotional or physical discomfort, whether it's tingling, tightness, pain, heat, or any sensation, the natural response may be to resist or suppress it. However, resisting these feelings can reinforce the blockage, making it harder to overcome.

Instead, the path to resolution involves embracing these sensations without judgment or the need to control them. By acknowledging and accepting what your body is feeling, you create space for the emotion to be processed and eventually fade away. Stay focused in your body while observing and experiencing the emotions with all bodily sensations with curiosity and openness.

Staying present with discomfort can be challenging but is essential for healing and personal growth. It allows you to unravel conditioned responses and unconscious patterns contributing to your subconscious blocks. Through this process, you develop resilience and inner strength, deepening your connection with yourself and your emotional experiences.

If these practices ever become too intense for you, you can stop. If you start to feel fearful, begin to shake or panic, please stop, look around the room you are in and then focus on one object. Let your system calm down. It is likely time to get help from a professional.

The goal is not to recreate a trauma response or relive anything traumatic. That would not be beneficial. You can touch into the emotions around anything in the past without reliving it. This practice is at clearing subconscious blocks and includes tuning into bodily sensations and allowing them to unfold naturally, rather than reacting defensively or trying to suppress them. Over time, this mindful approach can lead to profound insights and emotional release, paving the way for personal transformation and healing.

C is for Clear Meditation:

Begin by finding a quiet and comfortable space where you can sit undisturbed. Set an intention. What would you like to get out of your meditation? Close your eyes, allowing yourself to enter a state of inner stillness. With a straight spine and relaxed shoulders, place one hand on your lower abdomen, just below the navel, anchoring yourself in the present moment. As you inhale deeply, envision drawing in fresh, revitalizing energy, and as you exhale, imagine releasing any tension or blocked energy stored within.

As you engage in this practice, allow yourself to connect with any challenging emotions that may arise. If these emotions do not immediately surface, gently explore memories or physical sensations as starting points, gradually sinking deeper into the depths of your feelings. Remember, you don't have to relive past experiences entirely; simply acknowledging and touching into the emotions is often enough to initiate the flow of energy and facilitate release.

Practice the Full Breath, allowing each breath to carry you deeper into the layers of your subconscious mind. With each breath, allow yourself to sink into any physical sensations or emotions that arise for you. If nothing comes up, I suggest you think about your biggest problem and notice how you feel about it. Begin by breathing into that emotion. imagine yourself peeling away the layers of emotional armor, uncovering the raw, vulnerable emotions beneath. Stay with the strongest emotion until the intensity dissipates.

Trace the emotional track back to its origins, whether in infancy, childhood, or even prenatal stages. Use the full exhale to drift back in time, further and further back into your subconscious. Recognize that delving into these difficult emotions is a crucial step in the process of clearing stagnant energy that impedes your progress and clarity.

You want to get back to the deepest emotion that has been held in the subconscious. Once you get there, please stay with it, breathing into it and feeling it fully. How strong is it on a scale of one to ten? Notice how it feels in your body. Trust in the process, allowing yourself to move through each step at your own pace, knowing that healing unfolds in its own time.

<u>You don't have to completely re-live anything. You need to touch into the feelings just to get the energy flowing again</u>. By continuing to breathe into the emotion for as long as is required will activate and move the stuck energy and the block that is getting in the way for you. You want

to fully experience these difficult emotions until they clear. For example, 10-20 breaths into one emotion and it will start to shift.

If at any time your left brain kicks in and you start thinking all kinds of thoughts, just go back to the Full Breath. This usually happens when you stop breathing fully.

Once you breathe through one emotion, keep going and see if you can sink through it and touch into the emotion underneath.

Continue to follow the subconscious emotional track, without holding back.

Know that feeling into these difficult emotions helps clear the energy that is stuck in you and blocking you from moving forward and gaining clarity. Trust in the process. Keep going with this step until it feels complete. Moving into the next step too soon can limit the healing at this level. Don't rush and trust yourself in the timing.

The block or energetic space that you clear naturally fills itself with new, more uplifting emotions if you let it. Another way to fills the inner space you just cleared is by moving onto the empowerment stage.

As you continue to practice accessing and clearing your subconscious blocks through meditation and the Full Breath, remember that this journey is unique to you. Embrace each step with patience and compassion, knowing that every effort you make brings you closer to profound healing and personal growth.

Clarity offers numerous benefits that can transform our lives in profound ways. First, it provides focused direction, allowing us to set clear and specific goals. With a focused direction, we can channel our energy and resources efficiently to achieve these goals. Second, clarity enhances creativity by clearing subconscious blocks, unlocking our creative potential, and fostering innovative thinking and problem-solving abilities. Third, clarity brings inner peace. A clear mind and heart brings a sense of calm and confidence, freeing us from inner conflicts and uncertainties. Finally, clarity leads to greater fulfillment. By aligning our actions with our true desires, we experience deeper fulfillment and satisfaction in all aspects of life.

8

Empowerment - Reprogramming the Subconscious

"Believe in your infinite potential. Your only limitations are those you set upon yourself."

— *Roy T. Bennett*

Reprogramming the subconscious is a powerful tool for overcoming deep-seated issues and achieving true empowerment. By transforming limiting beliefs and healing deep traumas, you can unlock your full potential and live a more empowered life.

Testimonial: "Cheryl is who I call the 'Wound Healer.' I have referred to her people who have been grappling with the same trauma affecting their lives despite years of psychotherapy. Within a few sessions, she is able to do 'psychic surgery' and extract it from them providing insurmountable relief. She is nothing short of amazing. She has made a difference in many people's lives, including mine." —Dr. Achina Stein

This testimonial highlights Cheryl's exceptional ability to facilitate profound healing and reprogram the subconscious mind, offering insurmountable relief from long-standing trauma. It reinforces the transformative power of the techniques discussed in this chapter.

Now, let's dive into the most rewarding part of your journey. <u>This is where the power of deep breathing comes into play and helps rewire or reprogram the right side of your brain. The healing can be so profound that it feels as though past events never even happened</u>, allowing you to truly step into your greatness and live your soul's purpose.

Just to review, in the first step of ACCESS, we identify and acknowledge what the block is—the energy of trapped emotions due to wounding or trauma stuck within you. In the second step, CLEAR, we activate this energy by breathing into it and fully experiencing the associated emotions until they clear. During this process, the energetic space created often naturally fills itself. As we release old, challenging emotions, new and more uplifting feelings can emerge. Clearing significant blocks may take time, but it's a transformative journey.

In the EMPOWERMENT phase, we will reparent the younger self. This is the reprogramming step.

Reparenting your younger self is like becoming your own loving and supportive parent now, even for the child you once were. It involves giving yourself the care, understanding, and encouragement that you may not have received enough of when you were young. By doing this, you heal old wounds and build a stronger sense of self-love and security, paving the way to step into your greatness and live your soul's purpose.

Imagine if, when you were a child, you didn't always get the attention or reassurance you needed. Reparenting allows you to go back in your mind and heart to the time when your needs were not being met. By allowing yourself to become your younger self in your imagination, you can feel the feelings you couldn't process as a child. Children require their caregivers to be an emotional resource. When we didn't have that as a child, then our emotions become stuck because they haven't been processed. Once all the emotions are released, you can imagine yourself comforting that younger version of yourself. You might say kind and loving words you wish you had heard back then or give yourself the guidance and protection you longed for.

An example might be if your younger self felt neglected or unimportant because of busy or emotionally distant parents, visualize your present self giving your younger self a big, warm hug. Hear your present self saying, "You matter. Your feelings are important." This can replace old beliefs of feeling unworthy with new, empowering beliefs of being valued and significant.

"Feelings are much like waves, we can't stop them from coming but we can choose which ones to surf" -Jonatan Martensson

There are hundreds if not thousands of opportunities based on your childhood to practice this. Let's say you had a moment in school where you felt embarrassed or rejected by your peers. As your present self, visualize sitting beside your younger self at that moment, comforting them. Tell them, "It's okay to feel hurt. Your worth isn't determined by others' opinions." This process can help heal the emotional wounds from that experience and build your self-esteem.

The benefits of reparenting are profound. It can help you feel more confident and capable as an adult, knowing that you can provide for your own emotional needs. It also strengthens your inner resilience and self-worth, reducing the impact of past hurts on your present life. By reparenting, you create a nurturing environment within yourself where healing can happen, leading to greater happiness and healthier relationships.

Ultimately, reparenting your younger self is a way to reclaim your power and shape your future with compassion and understanding. It's about giving yourself the love and care you deserve, no matter what may have happened in the past. This practice allows you to grow into a more resilient and empowered person, ready to face life's challenges with greater strength and self-assurance, and fully capable of stepping into your greatness and living your soul's purpose.

Empowerment Medidtation

After moving through the ACCESS and CLEAR steps in the ACE Method, we will move into the EMPOWERMENT phase

Reparenting Your Younger Self: Imagine yourself as the adult you are today, silently or aloud telling your younger self everything they need to hear—assuring them they are loved, that it wasn't their fault, and so on. Breathe deeply and envelop your younger self in love, as if they were your cherished child. Offer the support and love that your younger self needed but didn't receive. Speak kindly to your inner child, saying things like, "You are loved," "You are safe," and "You are enough." This can help disarm any lingering feelings of self-blame and fill that part of you with unconditional love and acceptance.

Becoming Your Younger Self: Shift gears and visualize yourself at that younger age. Become the child you were. Breathe in the love and wisdom you've just received from your adult self. This process reprograms your subconscious and empowers you to embody your true self. Notice the emotions that arise as your younger self—do you feel loved, worthy? Acknowledge these feelings and breathe deeply to fully embrace the uplifting emotions. This back-and-forth communication will help reprogram your subconscious mind and reclaim your true power. Notice the emotions that come up—whether it's relief, joy, or even sadness.

Reflect: Take a moment to reflect on how this experience impacts your sense of self and well-being.

Return: Slowly bring your awareness back to the present moment. Wiggle your fingers and toes, stretch gently if needed. Open your eyes and take a final deep breath.

Continue connecting with your younger self in meditation over the next week or two to integrate these newfound emotions into your subconscious. Take some time every day to reconnect and breathe into the same uplifting emotions you experienced in your meditation.

I recommend starting with 10 or 20 minutes and working up to 45 minutes daily. Yes, that can be a stretch, but those who invest 45 minutes a day toward these meditations create significant change in their lives quickly.

Observe how this integration impacts your daily life. Over time, you may find yourself attracting different people and situations that align more closely with your authentic energy.

Commit to this practice for a week or two. Revisit your younger self daily, offering them the love and care they needed. Make these new, positive emotions a part of your subconscious. Imagine connecting with your inner child, offering the nurturing they missed out on, even before birth. This connection can lead to noticeable changes in your daily life. For example, you might find yourself more confident.

For example, you might have struggled with feeling not good enough in your job. After nurturing your inner child, you might start feeling more confident at work, leading to taking on new challenges and receiving positive feedback from colleagues and supervisors. This shift happens because you're now aligning with a stronger, more confident version of yourself.

A further example is that you may have often felt ignored as a child whenever you were upset. Practice visualizing your present self sitting with your inner child, listening to their worries, and saying, "I hear you, and your feelings are valid." As you integrate this, you might notice you start expressing your needs more clearly in your relationships now, and others respond more positively in social situations or more forgiving towards yourself when you make mistakes.

Find your own examples and you practice this, observe how these inner changes affect your everyday life. You may notice a transformation in the people you attract and the situations you find yourself in, aligning more closely with your authentic energy. Perhaps you start feeling more at peace in situations that used to trigger anxiety or find yourself attracting relationships that are supportive and understanding rather than critical.

In essence, clearing energetic subconscious blocks and reprogramming your subconscious in the empowerment phase is a profound journey of self-discovery and healing. It requires courage because fear is inevitable with this. It's scary and can be so challenging to feel your deepest difficult emotions. Patience is also required because it takes time. There is no single quick fix meditation that will heal and empower you completely. Self-compassion and self love are also necessary because you wouldn't be doing this if you received a lot of compassion and unconditional love when you were growing up. Do your best to give that to yourself now. By delving into your emotions and reclaiming your inner power, you pave the way for greater emotional well-being and personal growth. This process aligns you more closely with your true essence and purpose, leading to a more fulfilled and authentic life.

I will always remember when I met Becca through a chakra reading. Her energy felt unsettling, unlike anything I had encountered before. Instead of the usual flow of light and dark blocks in her chakras, it appeared as a haze of gray with scattered, diffuse bits of light here and there. I was deeply concerned for her well-being. Of all the hundreds of people I've done chakra readings for, I had never seen anything like it and still haven't seen it again to this day.

She shared with me that she was grappling with numerous health challenges, losing friends at a rapid pace, and had been in therapy for years. Above all, she felt lost and hopeless about life in general. She lacked direction and was struggling with depression. She was already in therapy and had been for a long time, but she had lost the will to live and nothing had been able to change that for her.

Despite these challenges, and the obvious lack of light in her being, I knew beyond a doubt that the Universe brought us together to do what was needed to help her rise to a whole new level of being. There was hope. I guided her through my 11-week program, helping her to uncover and release her most painful blocks, the stuck emotions held inside her for almost 70 years. She did the meditations and began to regain her inner strength and clarity.

We explored and healed early childhood issues and abuse through her marriage. She later admitted that when we met, she was considering taking her life as she felt utterly hopeless. Over time, she began to realize that her journey was about shining her inner light and embracing her creativity as an artist. She literally experienced shining her light and, at a group she began attending, was given the name Sparkie because of all her light. As she was breaking through from the darkness, she started writing a blog and continues to write that blog today, sharing her beautiful, profound perspective with the world in her own unique way.

Becca transformed her outlook from hopelessness to empowerment. Her health improved. She gained the clarity that she was meant to express herself through art. Today, she has emerged as a prolific artist and writer, inspiring others with her journey of healing and self-discovery. Through this process, Becca accessed her authentic power, allowing her inner light to shine brightly.

Her story is a powerful example of how clearing your subconscious blocks will help you find clarity and purpose and can bring light to even the darkest of times. It demonstrates the transformative power of healing and deep self-awareness, reminding us that with inner strength and guidance, we can navigate challenges and find our authentic power to live our true path in life.

By consistently applying the ACE Method, you will uncover deeper layers of your true self, paving the way for a life filled with clarity, empowerment, and fulfillment.

9

Developing Receptivity

"What helps me go forward is that I stay receptive, I feel that anything can happen."

— *Anouk Aimee*

Developing receptivity is a crucial aspect of your spiritual and energetic growth. It's about opening up and becoming more receptive with others, the world around you, and what wants to flow through you. If you find yourself giving and doing for others more than you are receiving, you are out of balance. Developing receptivity also means cultivating an openness to the subtle messages and energies that surround you, allowing them to guide and transform you.

In Western culture, many of us are taught to give more than we receive. An easy way to check in with yourself is to reflect on how well you receive compliments or offers of help. Do you often brush them off or take them in? For instance, when someone offers to assist you with a task or gives you a heartfelt compliment, do you graciously accept it, or do you instinctively decline or downplay it? This resistance to receiving can block the natural flow of energy and support that the Universe wants to provide for you.

Learning to receive is not about being selfish; it's about creating a harmonious balance where giving and receiving flow freely. By allowing yourself to be assisted and helped in return, you open up to greater abundance and connection. This balance is essential for your well-being and spiritual growth, as it nurtures both your inner and outer worlds.

I remember when I started dating my second husband, he would often give me compliments, and while I received them cognitively and somewhat emotionally, I realized one day that I didn't fully receive them. Yes, I moved beyond my old pattern of not receiving compliments and easily said, "thank you," and things like "that means a lot to me.", but I wasn't receiving his loving or kind words fully into my being. I became aware that I needed or truly wanted to level up my receiving. I told him what I noticed in the moment and asked him to repeat what he had just said. He happily went along with me and did so. This time I looked him in the eyes and said, "Thank You, Let Me Breathe That In." I stayed with the eye contact and took a few long breaths, focussing on the inhales, receiving his words and intention into my being. I was amazed at what I felt in my body. I continued to do this, and one of the wonderful benefits was that it made him feel appreciated at a deeper level.

I have taught this to many clients who need and want to develop better receptivity. One of my clients, Gini, leads retreats, and this is one of the practices she teaches. It is a common phrase now in her community. Maybe you would like to try this phrase with someone you feel close to. I encourage it!

Thinking of Gini, I'd like to share her story around developing receptivity. Gini was born to a heroin addict mother. You can only imagine how few of her needs were met. I found this out one day when I tuned into her energy flow and saw that she had a powerful expressive side but no energy at all in her receptive side. I started asking her questions about how this might play out in her life. She informed me that for as long as she could remember, her life was always about everyone else and she had to do her best to meet everyone else's needs. She didn't know how to fully receive anything that was offered to her, including and not limited to love, kindness, compliments, assistance, gifts, blessings, etc. Gini cried more than any other client, partly because she had so much grief. She had to grieve the life she never had since day one. She had to grieve not having her basic needs of connection and feeling loved and valued. We did some deep healing and empowerment around this and she loved the practice of receiving wherever she could and experienced some amazing personal shifts.

Receptivity is like developing a muscle that allows you to experience life with greater depth, understanding and fulfillment. My journey with receptivity expanded when, during the pandemic, my immigration from Canada to the US was put on hold. I had received approval to retrieve my belongings, but crossing the border was a challenge. Canada demanded people quarantine for 14 days. I just wanted my car. The American border patrol officers stated they didn't care if I quarantined or not. They suggested I just go across, get my car, and they'll let me back in. Well, I flew to Calgary and went through such an intense interrogation at the border, with people dressed like they were going to perform surgery and questioning me like I was a criminal. It was extremely intimidating. I was concerned that I had to answer a phone call daily for them to check in on me. I still had to get registration and insurance for my stored car in my brother's garage in Edmonton. The enormity of the situation set in. Sparing you the remainder of the details, I decided to quarantine in the hotel. I transferred to a larger room with a kitchen and bedroom. Emotionally overwhelmed and wondering what I was going to do, I decided to reschedule appointments on my calendar and create a personal meditation retreat for myself.

This is when I "received" the profound practice of surrender. I vividly remember sitting and trying to meditate, and I literally couldn't do it. I would get up and wander around, look out the window, or distract myself with various thoughts. I would try again, but to no avail. I even asked myself the magic question a few times. I couldn't believe what was happening. I have done countless retreats for myself and have led many people on personal retreats as well as group retreats. I was so frustrated, I went and sat on the bed with a few pillows behind my back so my back was at a 45-degree angle. I let myself feel the intensity of what I had been through. I asked God for help.

That's when it happened. I surrendered myself and my situation to the Universe. I started to cry and didn't stop until all the tears had flowed. I used the Full Breath as I am so accustomed to deep release from the subconscious. I opened up and began to feel myself as being held. This was all meant to be this way. I was loved and cared for, and I received Universal love and caring in every cell of my being. I moved deeply into knowing that something good was going to come from this. This profound experience was a turning point, allowing me to step into my greatness and live my soul's purpose with renewed clarity and strength. I had to receive the retreat. It wasn't me guiding it. I opened up and received all the Universe wanted to give. I am eternally grateful for all the blessings of that powerful retreat.

The process of unlearning and surrender plays a profound role in deepening one's connection to inner wisdom and universal consciousness. Often, we accumulate beliefs, habits, and conditioning throughout our lives that limit our understanding of ourselves and the world around us. Spiritual unlearning involves shedding these layers of conditioning to uncover our true essence and innate wisdom. Surrender, on the other hand, entails letting go of the ego's need for control and opening up to not being in charge. Then you can move into trusting in the divine flow of life. Together, these practices open pathways to profound spiritual transformation and alignment with higher truths.

Spiritual unlearning begins with introspection, self-awareness, and developing receptivity. It requires a willingness to question deeply held beliefs and societal norms that may no longer serve our highest good. This process invites us to examine our conditioning with honesty and compassion, acknowledging how these beliefs shape our perceptions and behaviors. Through these practices of developing receptivity and surrender, you can uncover unconscious patterns and thought structures that inhibit our spiritual growth. Being receptive to new insights and perspectives as well as that the fact that we are always loved, supported and guided is crucial in this journey of self-discovery.

Unlearning involves releasing attachments to identities and narratives that define us but may not align with our authentic self. It requires embracing vulnerability and openness to new perspectives, allowing space for personal evolution and spiritual expansion. By relinquishing outdated beliefs and embracing a mindset of curiosity and exploration, we create room for deeper spiritual insights and transformative experiences. Developing receptivity to these new insights can help us navigate this process more effectively, fostering a sense of openness and readiness for change.

Surrender is a cornerstone of spiritual practice, inviting us to relinquish the illusion of control and surrender to divine love and intelligence guiding our lives. It involves trusting in the greater wisdom of the Universe and accepting life's uncertainties with grace and equanimity. Surrender does not imply passivity but rather an active engagement with the present moment, free from resistance and attachment to outcomes.

Through surrender, we cultivate inner peace and resilience, recognizing that challenges and obstacles are opportunities for growth and learning. It fosters humility and gratitude, allowing us to embrace life's experiences as valuable lessons on our spiritual journey. Surrendering involves letting go of the ego's desires and expectations, opening ourselves to divine guidance and intuitive wisdom that transcends the limitations of the rational mind. By being receptive to this guidance, we can more easily align with the unconditional love, higher truths and wisdom that flow from the divine.

In summary, the practices of spiritual unlearning and surrender are deeply interconnected with the development of receptivity. By unlearning, we clear the space within ourselves to receive new, higher truths. By surrendering, we trust and remain open to the flow of the divine at all levels. Together, these practices lead to profound spiritual growth, inner peace, and a deeper alignment with our true selves, our authentic power and the power of the Universe.

Developing receptivity also involves being attuned to the environment around you. The Universe constantly communicates with us through our surroundings, offering guidance and support in subtle ways. For instance, recently on a walk, I encountered a series of goose feathers, seemingly out of nowhere. Despite having never felt drawn to that particular area before, I sensed a profound message from the Universe:

a reminder to be open to new paths and experiences. It was also provided for me to teach this to a group of women in one of my programs.

Such signs and symbols are the Universe's way of aligning you with your highest self. Everything in our environment carries a vibration, and by being receptive, you can discern which vibrations are beneficial for your growth and well-being. This ongoing dialogue with the Universe requires you to remain open and aware, trusting that the messages you receive are guiding you toward greater alignment and harmony.

In my workshops, I've witnessed how developing receptivity can lead to profound physical and energetic cleansing. For example, several women experienced diarrhea immediately prior to the day of an on-line session—a symbolic release of what no longer served them. This physical manifestation was a form of energetic purging, making way for new, higher vibrations to enter their lives. It happened that I was introducing a new, powerful practice that would lift them to a higher vibration in their bodies and toward becoming more of their true authentically powerful selves.

I still enjoy an old Sufi prayer, which I love to sing over and over or sometimes breathe to in meditation for a long time. It cleanses me of all my perceived expectations of who and what I should be. It takes me out of uncertainty and into knowing. It helps me surrender to and receive the love and compassion of the Universe. It helps me completely surrender to trust and faith.

> *Take Me Just the Way I AM*
> *Summon All I'm Meant to Be*
> *Place Your Seal Upon My Heart*
> *And Live in Me*

A critical aspect of developing receptivity is understanding and transcending the illusion of separation. In our daily lives, we often perceive ourselves as separate from others—our partners, friends, and even the aspects of ourselves we dislike. However, this perceived separation is merely an illusion. In truth, we are all interconnected, part of a greater whole.

By recognizing this interconnectedness, you can move beyond feelings of isolation and embrace the oneness that binds us all. This realization helps you become more receptive to the energies and messages from others and the Universe. The feathers I encountered serve as symbols of this unity, helping us release what no longer serves and inviting new, higher vibrations into our lives.

Sometimes, developing receptivity means letting go of old practices and being open to new ways of experiencing and understanding the world. I recall an encounter with a BriBri shaman whom I had met in Costa Rica. We spoke through a translator and he was delighted by my curiosity about the work he did. One day he appeared to me in meditation and began teaching me a practice to increase my spiritual power. I went with it. But when I returned to my traditional shamanic practices, he made me very sick. I discovered this when out of desperation, I called a shamanic friend who healed me of this. The Bri Bri shaman didn't want me to do any other practices other than his. At the time, I was deeply attached to my practice of journeying through a cedar tree and resisted giving it up. In hindsight, I realize that my reluctance to release my old methods prevented me from fully embracing a potentially powerful new way of receiving guidance.

This missed opportunity taught me the importance of being willing to let go of familiar practices or ways of being and open myself to new possibilities. By surrendering my attachment to my old way of journeying, I could have accessed deeper levels of healing and insight offered by the shaman's telepathic work. Still, making someone sick seems mean to me.

Years later when I joined a spiritual school, I wanted to fully open up to and embrace the new practices I was learning. I let go of the shamanic drum I had made years earlier and gave away my rattle. I never regretted it. Even though I had let go of shamanic practices, my power animals still returned to me when I needed them most.

A classic practice of surrender used by many in 12 step programs is "Let Go and Let God".

This practice encourages one to develop energetic receptivity. This is an ongoing journey that requires you to cultivate an open and flexible mindset. By embracing surrender, tuning into the messages from the Universe, and overcoming the illusion of separation, you can align more deeply with your true self and the higher vibrations that support your growth. Remember, receptivity is not about passivity but about actively engaging with the energies and guidance around you in a state of openness and trust. As you continue to develop this essential muscle, you will find yourself more attuned to the subtle currents of the Universe, allowing them to guide and transform you in profound ways.

Developing Receptivity Meditation

Sit up straight with the top of your head lifted toward the ceiling. Stretch your shoulders up and back. Then let them fall naturally. Feel your feet on the floor and your seat firmly on the chair. Shift around slightly to bring full awareness into your body. Take a deep breath, focusing on your lower abdomen. Make your breath rhythmic, syncing it with your heartbeat or pulse. Use the words "love" and "light" to go into your root chakra

Root Chakra (Safety and Stability)
As you inhale, visualize unconditional love from the Earth rising through your feet to your heart. Then exhale this energy down through your body and out your feet. Feel supported by Mother Earth. Call in your spiritual support and breathe deeply, focusing on your root chakra. Breathe love and light into this chakra, imagining the energy coming in from the left and flowing out to the right. This balances the left, feminine side, and right, masculine side of your energy. If you feel any resistance, breathe through it, widening the stream of love and light until you feel stable and secure. Continue with this until you experience a sense of increased safety and/or stability.

Sacral Chakra (Creativity and Passion)
Move your focus to your sacral chakra, located a few inches below your navel, near the spine. Inhale love and light from the left, and exhale it to the right. This chakra is linked to creativity, passion, and relationships. Feel the energy as you breathe, filling up this area. Widen the stream of energy, allowing it to flow freely. If emotions arise, breathe through them,

allowing the energy to cleanse any pain or blockages. Continue until you feel inspired, connected, creative, etc.

Solar Plexus Chakra (Personal Power and Truth)
Focus on your solar plexus, located just below the sternum. This chakra governs personal power and truth. Inhale love and light from the left, nurturing your sense of personal power, and exhale love and light to the right. Notice how the energy flows, perhaps holding it in the chakra before expressing it outwards. Widen the stream of energy if it feels correct, enhancing your clarity and alignment with your truth. Continue with this until you feel more light and/or have uncovered a hidden truth.

Heart Chakra (Love and Compassion)
Move your awareness to your heart chakra in the center of your chest. Inhale love and light from the left, receiving the abundance of the Universe, and exhale it to the right. Focus on receiving and expressing love and compassion. Widen the flow, opening up the chakra to a large stream, allowing yourself to feel deeply connected and loved.

Throat Chakra (Expression of Truth)
Focus on your throat chakra, located in the middle of your neck. Breathe in love and light, allowing yourself to express your true self. Inhale from the left and exhale to the right, expanding the flow of energy. Widen the stream to include your shoulders, jaw, and ears, imagining the energy flowing through and revitalizing your throat chakra. Continue with this until you feel a new sense of confidence in speaking your truth or, at the highest level, expressing your purpose.

Place your hands on your heart. Breathe normally and reflect on the experience. Think about which chakras felt significant and what you want to focus on in the future. Write down your thoughts in a journal to revisit and deepen your practice.

As you continue your journey of spiritual and energetic growth, remember that developing receptivity is not just a practice but a way of life. By opening yourself to the subtle messages and energies around you, you allow the Universe to guide and support you in ways you may have never imagined. Embrace the balance of giving and receiving, and recognize that allowing yourself to receive is a vital part of your journey toward wholeness. Trust in the process, surrender to the flow, and know that each step you take brings you closer to your true, powerful self. Your capacity to receive is directly linked to your ability to manifest your deepest desires and live a life of fulfillment and joy. Stay open, stay receptive, and let the magic unfold.

10

Are You a Hole Filler?

"The only people who get upset about you setting boundaries are the ones who were benefiting from you having none."

— *Anonymous*

What is a hole filler? See if you recognize yourself or others in this story. I once had a friend who I spoke with frequently. We lived quite a distance from each other so we only got together in person periodically. We seemed to have a lot in common at the beginning of the friendship and enjoyed each other's company. Over time, like in any relationship, I started to see some of her true colors which were not so appealing. They slowly surfaced and I would look at them with compassion and the attitude that nobody's perfect. Then some bigger things started presenting and I soon made me realize that the friendship seemed out of balance.

It consistently seemed to be much more about her and not about me. I clearly had a deeper layer in me that wanted to be healed.

I had a good friend back in Canada who used to say, all your friends are allowed to have three faults. If they start to have more than that, you might want to start questioning the relationship. When I look at my decades-long friendships, none of them have more than three faults and it's not even about counting them. A part of me wanted to end the friendship as I didn't have much hope. With this friend, when I tried talking about concerns when I had them in the past, I was responded to with denial and defensiveness. Nothing resolved. I didn't feel heard nor understood. I decided to tune into her energetically and immediately saw that she had a black hole in the center of her heart chakra - and she wanted me to fill it! Wow! That's not my job I thought. I don't want to be a hole filler. And I'm certain you don't want to be one either.

I asked myself, as I always do, what is this reflecting back to me? What do I have to learn here? How does this serve me? I realized it had nothing to do with her. I had wanted to step away from the friendship a number of times and it was my husband who convinced me to not do that, thinking he was being a good husband. I gave my power over to my husband. Uggh. When I talked to him about it later, he completely understood. And, it's still my responsibility to always do what is in my highest good, because that will always be in the highest good of all.

I cannot know her soul's journey. I wish her all the love and blessings on her path. After I let her go, new women who aligned more closely with who I am began to enter my life. The shift was startling, and I embraced every bit of it.

Many of my clients often say they put everyone else first or that they come in last in their lives. You can't start putting yourself first until you stop filling other people's holes. The holes that people have are unmet needs from childhood. They weren't loved enough, listened to enough and naturally, continued on in life trying to fill that empty space through others, not realizing they are the ones that need to fill that hole through loving and caring for themselves. At some point in their life, it felt like they had to "earn" love or that their needs don't matter, so they put other people's needs first.

Setting boundaries can profoundly impact your relationships and personal well-being. Take Sarah, for instance, who constantly found herself overwhelmed at work because she never said no. Her colleagues would regularly offload their tasks onto her, knowing she would always agree to help. This led to burnout and a lack of time for her own responsibilities. Realizing the toll it was taking on her, Sarah decided to set clear boundaries. She started to politely but firmly decline additional tasks, explaining that she needed to focus on her own workload. Initially, some colleagues were taken aback, but over time, they began to respect her boundaries. As a result, Sarah experienced less stress, improved productivity, and regained control over her work-life balance.

Similarly, consider Jane, who struggled with family dynamics during holidays. Every year, her relatives would expect her to host large gatherings, despite her limited space and busy schedule. Feeling obligated, Jane complied, which left her exhausted and resentful. One year, Jane chose to set boundaries by clearly communicating her limitations. She suggested alternative plans, like rotating hosting duties among family members or meeting at a more convenient location. While some family members were resistant at first, Jane's consistency in maintaining her boundaries eventually led to more equitable arrangements. This allowed Jane to enjoy the holidays without the undue pressure, fostering healthier family interactions and a more balanced personal life.

These examples illustrate that while setting boundaries can be challenging and may initially meet resistance, the long-term benefits of reduced stress, improved relationships, and enhanced well-being are well worth the effort.

In his book "When the Body Says No," Gabor Maté explores how chronic illness can be linked to early lack of attachment with the mother. When we enter the world and do not develop a strong connection to our mother, the result is that we often fill emotional voids or become co-dependent on others. It's important to understand that this isn't anyone's fault. Many mothers in the past didn't know about the benefits of oxytocin which is the bonding hormone released from eye contact with their baby or the necessity of skin-to-skin contact with them. Oxytocin is essential for forming strong, loving attachments.

He also had done a great deal of research on people with ALS. Lou Gehrig's name is associated with ALS (Amyotrophic Lateral Sclerosis). Gehrig's personality of selflessness and extreme helpfulness fits what Dr. Gabor Maté believes is common among ALS patients. Gehrig experienced childhood trauma because he grew up with an alcoholic parent.

Gabor Maté's research shows a strong link between chronic illness and the denial of one's emotional needs. He argues that people who ignore their feelings or prioritize others' needs over their own are more likely to develop serious health issues. According to Maté, this suppression of emotions can stress the body and weaken the immune system, making individuals more vulnerable to chronic illnesses.

People pleasing can lead to giving away one's power and losing one's sense of self. As you undergo internal shifts and realign your energy patterns, expressing these changes becomes essential in all aspects of life. This involves setting both internal and external boundaries. Internally, it means establishing limits and respecting your own emotions, thoughts, and needs. Externally, it requires clearly communicating and upholding your boundaries and expectations in relationships and interactions.

By setting these boundaries, you honor your inner world while safeguarding your personal space. Boundary setting not only preserves your emotional and mental well-being but also supports ongoing self-development. Embracing boundaries allows you to focus on your goals with renewed confidence, ensuring that your external environment aligns with your internal growth. This also contributes to a more harmonious and fulfilling life.

To me, this is a life's work and is so worthwhile. Once we have strong, healthy boundaries, we can be confident in all situations. This confidence is part of our true inner power. Here is a simplified meditation to help you end people pleasing and do the healing required to easily and automatically set healthy boundaries without even having to think twice about it.

Meditation to End People Pleasing

1. *Relax: Sit up straight, close your eyes, and take long, full, deep breaths. Feel the chair beneath you, holding and supporting you.*
2. *Sacred Space: Once you are in the flow of the Full Breath, imagine being in a sacred space, surrounded by spiritual support. Call upon this support to help you clear blocks and embrace the importance of putting yourself first when appropriate.*
3. *Breath Focus: Breathe deeply, engaging your abdominal muscles. Inhale for a count of 6-8 seconds, then exhale for a count of 6-8. Focus on the emotions tied to people-pleasing and not putting yourself first.*
4. *Root Chakra: Bring your eyes down to your root chakra. It is at the tip of your tailbone. Continue breathing fully and notice any physical sensations or emotions. Breathe into any emotions that come up, trusting the Full Breath is releasing them.*

5. *Revisit the Past: Allow yourself to drift back in time, likely to early childhood or the moment when these emotions first began. Become your younger self and feel those emotions deeply, continuing to breathe into them. Acknowledge any subconscious beliefs formed during this time, such as "I am..." and "People are...".*

   Here are some examples to help you identify these beliefs:

   - *"I am bad."*
   - *"I am unworthy."*
   - *"I am not good enough."*
   - *"I am unlovable."*
   - *"I am sad."*

   Similarly, consider beliefs about others:

   - *"People are untrustworthy."*
   - *"People are judgmental."*
   - *"People are indifferent."*
   - *"People are unkind."*

   As you breathe into these derogatory subconscious beliefs, allow yourself to fully experience them without judgment. Recognize their presence and the impact they've had on your life. With each breath, imagine releasing these beliefs and creating space for new, empowering truths.

6. *Release and Affirm: As your younger self, hear these affirmations: "None of this was your fault.*

You were worthy of being number one. You deserve to feel like you matter." Breathe in these truths deeply.
7. *Adult Self: Shift to your adult self. Imagine picking up and comforting your younger self, affirming their worth and importance. Share with them all the truths about being number one when appropriate.*
8. *New Beliefs: Form new beliefs about yourself, others, and love. "I feel...", "People are...", "Love and caring is...". Breathe these new truths into your root chakra.*
9. *Daily Demonstration: Ask your adult self how they can demonstrate daily that you are number one. Make a commitment to prioritize your needs and emotions.*
10. *Seal and Finish: Seal these affirmations into your root chakra. When ready, open your eyes and feel grounded in your new understanding of self-worth.*

As we conclude this chapter, remember that setting boundaries and prioritizing your needs is not an act of selfishness but one of self-respect and self-love. By recognizing and addressing the patterns of being a "hole filler," you empower yourself to create healthier, more balanced relationships. Embrace this journey of self-discovery and growth, knowing that it leads to a more fulfilling and authentic life. May you continue to honor your inner power and cultivate the strength to put yourself first, paving the way for deeper connections and true well-being.

11

New Beginnings

"The magic in new beginnings is truly the most powerful of them all."
— *Josiyah Martin*

We are now moving into new beginnings and the importance of embracing change. New beginnings are vital for growth and allow us to start over. I once knew a remarkable therapist named Leanne Hartley. I attended her Hakomi body-centered psychotherapy workshops, where she would often say, "You can always start over."

This idea of beginning again resonates deeply with me. To truly start anew, we must first identify and release what no longer serves us. This might involve relationships, careers, studies, retirement, motherhood, health, or spirituality. Reflecting on what feels out of place or unfulfilling is crucial. Often, our environment mirrors what needs to be released and healed—whether it's an attitude, an old wound, or something else blocking our progress.

Many people wait until New Year's Eve to set new intentions, but we can choose to start over at any time. While visions and goals are valuable, we often limit our imagination of what's possible. We are more powerful than we realize, and I will repeat my saying on being powerful. Please receive this: You Are Powerful Beyond Belief, Powerful Beyond What You Can Imagine. Embracing new beginnings allows you to open up to setting goals and embracing visions without having to know exactly what it is or being constrained by our human expectations. Our best visions often come through meditation, receptivity, and realization.

A notable example is my client Gini Trask, who realized her calling as a spiritual leader through our work together, despite initial resistance. Here's what she had to say after the first time we worked together: "I had built a seven-figure business, I was so burnt out, and so exhausted, because the business that I had, basically reinforced my issues around 'receiving.' The clients that I had actually, literally, beat me down on price constantly. With Cheryl, I have come through the dark night of the soul. It has been hard, but there's been a lot of releasing of old patterns. Now I have this totally different bright future. Yes, I walked away from a seven-figure business, but I also walked away from reinforcing old patterns and old beliefs that don't work for me - all of those blocks that were holding me back. And the future is just so bright. I've stepped into who I really am, instead of who I thought I had to be. I have discovered I am a spiritual leader, and even though I resisted that initially, I now embrace it. I've changed my career and attract the right people and the right clients and, and get paid really well. All of that through your program. So it's been fantastic." - Gini Trask

Supporting your new beginning with symbols can be very effective. Symbols work at the conscious and subconscious levels and will assist you in creating the new beginning that is ideal for where you are at.

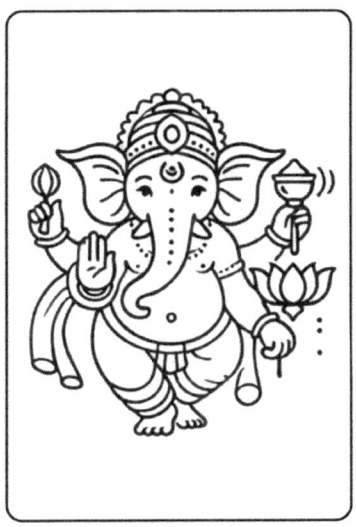

One powerful symbol is Ganesh, an ancient Hindu deity revered as the remover of obstacles and a patron of new beginnings. Ganesh's story, involving his birth and transformation, reflects the theme of overcoming difficulties to start anew. Attuning to Ganesh can help align your energy with new beginnings and removing obstacles. You might keep an image, statue, or other representations of Ganesh to meditate on and inspire your journey.

Another meaningful symbol is the lotus flower, often depicted at the base of Ganesh. The lotus represents purity and rebirth, rising from the mud to bloom beautifully, symbolizing new beginnings.

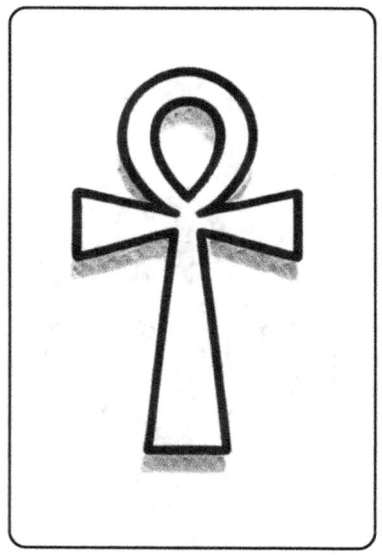

The Ankh is another powerful symbol of new life and renewal. Originating in Egypt, the Ankh signifies regeneration and starting over. It is a powerful ancient Egyptian symbol that can guide you on your journey through life and beyond. It is a simple yet profound design—a cross with a loop at the top and carries deep meanings that resonate across time. The shape and design are most symbolic. Picture the Ankh as a cross with an oval loop at the top. This loop, or "handle," represents the key to life. The vertical line stands for your path in life, and the crossbar symbolizes the connection between your earthly experiences and the divine. This elegant symbol captures the essence of both the material world and eternal spiritual life. Think of the loop as representing eternal life or the soul's journey beyond physical existence. It symbolizes infinity and the boundless nature of your spiritual self. The crossbar and vertical line reflect your life's journey and how it intersects with higher spiritual truths. Together, these elements remind you of the connection between your everyday life and your eternal soul.

Bring the Ankh symbol into your life by using it as a personal symbol to guide you toward renewal and a deeper understanding of your life's journey. Let it remind you of your eternal soul and the connections that bind all of life.

Try meditating with a physical Ankh talisman right in front of you, or maybe you want to hold it in your hand. I have even tucked it into my bra to have it close to my heart. You can also imagine it by visualizing its shape, color, and texture. Open up to it and let it help you focus on your spiritual essence and life force. Meditating on the Ankh can help you release old patterns and embrace new beginnings.

You can easily incorporate the Ankh into your daily life. Whether you wear it as jewelry, display it in your home, or keep a small image with you, the Ankh can serve as a constant reminder of your purpose and spiritual path, whether you know what that is or not, still trusting that you are going through internal growth and this is a new beginning.

In summary, the Ankh is more than a symbol; it's a guide to understanding life's eternal nature and your place within it. By embracing the Ankh, you connect with a tradition that honors life, renewal, and the profound balance of existence.

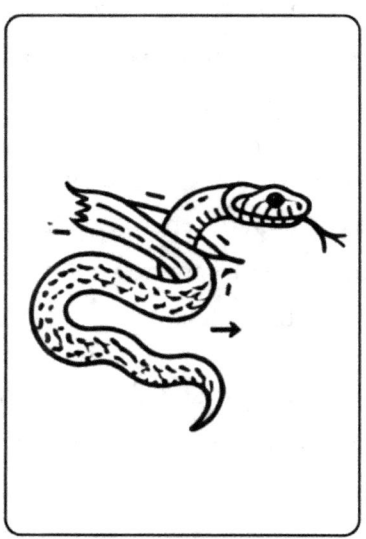

A somewhat unexpected symbol for me, and yet one of my favorites, is snake. Specifically, the albino Burmese python is dear to me. The snake symbolizes a powerful new beginning because of its ability to shed its skin, releasing the past and embracing renewal. When a snake sheds its skin, it undergoes a transformative process, letting go of the old and emerging rejuvenated. It enters a trance-like state, shedding its old skin as if reborn.

Ted Andrews writes at length about the snake in his book *Animal Speak*. This was my first spiritual book. He states the snake is about transformation and rebirth, healing and medicine, intuition and wisdom, and more.

Perhaps you've come across a discarded snake skin in nature, witnessing this symbolic act firsthand. Even if snakes aren't your favorite creatures, their symbolism remains potent. I used to be afraid of snakes, but through meditation, I came to appreciate their symbolism of transformation and new beginnings.

If you are interested, there is a snake shedding meditation in my first book, *Heal Your Neck Issues and Let Your Throat Chakra Shine*. You can certainly contact me and ask me for the recording. Remember, seeing a snake in nature is likely the sign of the Universe supporting you in embarking on a new beginning.

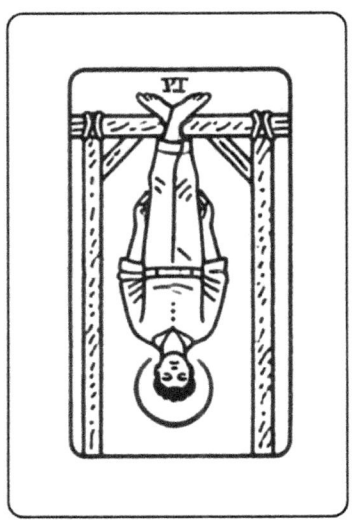

In Tarot, the Hanged Man card symbolizes a change in perspective. It invites us to let go of old judgments and views, opening up to new ways of seeing situations, people, and ourselves. The Hanged Man Tarot Card is often associated with themes of surrender, sacrifice, suspension, new perspective, and letting go. The Hanged Man card typically depicts a man hanging upside down by one foot from a tree or a wooden frame. Despite his inverted position, he often appears serene or even enlightened, with a halo around his head, symbolizing spiritual awakening and enlightenment. This tarot card, with its call for surrender and new perspectives, can be a powerful reminder to embrace the flow of life, along with its beginnings and change. Open yourself up to meditate with Hanged Man, turning yourself upside down to gain new perspectives and let go of what no longer serves you. Incorporating these symbols into your life, perhaps on an altar or in a personal space, can serve as subconscious reminders of your commitment to starting over. An altar doesn't have to be elaborate; it can be as simple or as intricate as you like. It's a place to focus your energy and intentions daily.

I will hold you in my heart as you embark on your new beginning. I have put this energy into this book if you choose to receive it. Embrace this time of transformation and growth, and remember that starting over is an act of reclaiming your innate power. May Ganesh, the Ankh, snake, and the Hanged Man guide you towards a fresh, empowered start.

Let's explore the theme of new beginnings and the power they hold to transform our lives. This guided meditation will help you embrace change, release what no longer serves you, and open yourself to new possibilities.

New Beginnings Meditation

Let's start by finding a comfortable position, sitting nice and straight with your feet on the floor. Close your eyes, relax your body. The Universe is holding you through the chair you sit in. When you're ready, begin breathing with the Full Breath, allowing yourself to settle into this moment.

Step 1: Releasing What No Longer Serves You

Imagine your life in general right now and breathe into it, exactly as it is. Notice what comes up. It could be something in your relationships, career, studies, or even your role in retirement or motherhood. Reflect on your health and spirituality too. How does it feel? Are there any emotions that want to be felt that you wouldn't allow previously? Trust your emotions around what comes up and breathe into them for some time. This begins the releasing of what no longer serves you. The trapped emotions inside you are holding people, things, and situations that are no longer in your highest good. Notice what the emotions are attached to. What do you need to let go of to make room for a new beginning? What feels heavy or outdated?

What chakra(s) are these attached to? Or maybe you notice the emotion at some point in your body. I invite you to release whatever has a hold on you by imagining a waterfall coming down over you and through you.

Inhale through your nose and silently out your mouth with long breaths. On the inhale, breathe into whatever needs to be released and on the exhale, feel it washing away, down into the earth. Feel them wash away, leaving you feeling lighter and more free.

You may want to repeat this section again and again before moving on to the next portions.

Step 2: Embracing Symbols of New Beginnings

Let's connect with the symbols that represent new beginnings and resonate with you. It is usually best to focus on one and open up to that one symbol supporting you in the most powerful ways.

1. Ganesh – The Remover of Obstacles
Visualize Ganesh, the beloved Hindu deity. He stands before you, his elephant head wise and compassionate. Feel his energy, ready to help clear your path of obstacles. Bring him into your heart chakra. Ask Ganesh what he brings you and see what happens, allowing him to radiate all that he is inside your being.

2. The Ankh – Symbol of Life and Renewal Next, envision the Ankh, an ancient Egyptian symbol. See its looped cross shape glowing with vitality. As you hold it in your hand, feel its connection to life and renewal. Let it remind you of the continuous cycle of beginnings and endings, and the opportunity for rebirth. Imagine bringing it into your heart chakra and let it fill you with vibrant energy, renewing your spirit and opening you to new possibilities in your new life.

3. Snake – Shedding the Past and Rebirth Now, picture a snake shedding its skin. It symbolizes the release of old patterns and the emergence of something new. Imagine yourself shedding your old skin, leaving behind what no longer serves you. Feel yourself becoming lighter, ready to embrace a fresh start with clarity and strength.

4. The Hanged Man – New Perspectives Finally, visualize the Hanged Man from the Tarot, hanging upside down. This symbolizes letting go of old perspectives to see things in a new light. Picture yourself adopting a fresh view of your life, opening up to new possibilities and understanding. Allow yourself to see your situations, people, and purpose from this new perspective, ready to embrace the change with open arms.

Step 3: Integrating Your New Beginning

Breathe deeply and feel the energy of your symbol integrating into your being. Ganesh clears your path, the Ankh revitalizes you, snake helps you shed the old and rebirth, and the Hanged Man offers new perspectives. Visualize yourself stepping into this new beginning, feeling lighter and freer. Embrace the excitement and potential of what's ahead.

As you prepare to return to your day, take a moment to express gratitude for this journey. Know that these symbols are always with you, guiding and supporting you in your path of renewal. Gently bring your awareness back to the present moment. Wiggle your fingers and toes, take a deep breath, and when you're ready, open your eyes. Welcome to your new beginning. You have the power to start over, to create, and to become your greatest self.

As we reach the end of this chapter on new beginnings, remember that the power to start anew lies within you. Embrace change, release what no longer serves you, and open yourself to the boundless possibilities that lie ahead. Trust in the process and the symbols that guide you—Ganesh, the Ankh, the snake, and the Hanged Man—as you step into a fresh, empowered start. You are powerful beyond belief, and each new beginning is a testament to your strength and potential. Welcome this time of transformation with an open heart and mind, knowing that you are on the path to becoming your greatest self.

12
Healing and Empowerment to True Purpose

"The privilege of a lifetime is to become who you truly are."
— Carl Jung

Healing and empowerment are intrinsically linked to discovering and living your true purpose. Through the process of clearing deep subconscious blocks, you can access a more authentic and powerful version of yourself, enabling you to align with your soul's purpose.

Testimonial: "When I first started to work with Cheryl, I was just ready to start my speaking career again, and my biggest challenge at that time was attracting clients, the right group of people to help me and to start paid speaking gigs. Cheryl's tremendous genius in her work, guidance, and direction took me deeper with traumas than I even knew I had. It was deeper than 40 years of psychotherapy and other trauma modalities I had done. Cheryl is

very kind, empathetic, and really is there for you. I'm attracting helpful people now and getting support for my speaking business and seminars. I would say to anyone who is ready to take the next step in their life and is willing to be brave and go very deep to have the kind of 'well-being' in yourself to blossom your life, Cheryl is the one for you. I am most grateful to have met someone who is gifted and able to see things I felt but couldn't pinpoint, and now we are right in the root of issues to melt and heal them. This is a beginning I've waited for my whole life."
—Vicki Mizel

This testimonial illustrates the transformative power of healing and how it can propel you toward your true purpose. Vicki's experience highlights the deep work involved and the profound impact it can have on all areas of life.

My own healing journey started over 30 years ago when I was on the beach with a friend who was doing kinesiology on me. It was a gorgeous day on Vancouver Island, and we were waiting for the tide to go out so we could pick oysters. She was doing some energetic clearing on me and kept naming family members with whom energy was attached. I'll never forget being there on the beach. Listening to her speak, the ocean waves hit the shore in the background when suddenly a huge ball of white light with the most intense love I have ever felt, hovered over me. I knew beyond a shadow of a doubt that it was my younger brother who had taken his life a couple years earlier. I kept waiting for her to mention him. Finally, she did and said, "He is here." And I said, "I know." Neither of us had ever experienced the presence of a spirit before.

He spoke to me through her, and his message was to start meditating. He had taken his life a year and a half before that and told us he was bipolar, which had not been diagnosed. I started meditating and within a few months healed my own depression. I didn't know I was becoming my own energy healer, but I healed my tinnitus, chronic neck and shoulder pain, and a tremendous amount of emotional wounding.

Healing and empowerment are not just processes; they are profound explorations that invite you to step into your greatness and live your soul's purpose. I never fully realized my own adventurous spirit until I took the leap—selling all I had and setting out to explore the world. Indeed, the journey of personal growth itself is a profound exploration, full of twists, turns, and discoveries for those bold enough to embark upon it.

Every great journey begins with a call. Sometimes it's a whisper during the quiet moments of your day, a sense that there's more to life than what you're currently experiencing. Other times, it's a loud, unmistakable pull—a job loss, a relationship ending, or a health crisis that leaves you with no choice but to seek something new. This call is the first step in your journey of healing, empowerment, and discovering your true purpose.

My own call came at a pivotal moment. I was comfortable and successful by societal standards, yet I felt a profound emptiness. Some may have viewed it as the spark of adventure, but the longing to slow down coupled with the longing for something more—had always been there. It wasn't until I decided to listen and to act, that my true journey began. The decision to sell every material thing I owned and step into the unknown wasn't easy, but it felt necessary. It marked the beginning of a transformative process that would reshape my understanding of myself and my place in the world.

Answering the call to personal change means leaving behind the familiar and stepping into the unknown. This can be terrifying. We often cling to what we know, even if it's unfulfilling, because it feels safe. Yet, safety can also mean stagnation. Embracing the journey of healing and empowerment requires courage and the willingness to face our fears and uncertainties, knowing that each step brings us closer to living our soul's purpose.

For me, leaving my comfort zone was a mixture of excitement and trepidation. I had to confront my fears of the unknown. My friends, family, clients, neighbors would ask me if I was scared. Yes, I would have moments of intense fear. What did I think I was doing? And whenever that fear arose, I would just sit myself down and breathe through it. Then I could return to the strong knowing in my heart. It was the fear of the unknown, of going to developing countries where I didn't speak the language that would surface. But with each step, I discovered new strengths within myself—abilities I never knew I had. The journey was teaching me that healing isn't about escaping pain but about confronting it and transforming it into something meaningful.

Each challenge became an opportunity to step into more of my authentic power.

As you embark on your journey from blocked to powerful, you'll find that the path of healing and empowerment is not linear. It's a winding road filled with both challenges and triumphs. Along the way, you'll encounter obstacles that test your resolve and moments of clarity that illuminate your path. These moments of clarity are crucial because they provide a deeper understanding of your true self and align you with your purpose.

In my journey, I traveled to numerous countries, lived with indigenous tribes, and immersed myself in diverse cultures. These experiences were more than just physical adventures; they were profound opportunities for growth and learning. Living with the Maasai in Kenya and the Shuar in Ecuador, I was not just exploring new places, people and cultures, I was also uncovering hidden parts of myself. The simplicity and depth of their lives taught me about resilience, community, and the power of purpose. Each experience added a new layer to my understanding of healing and empowerment, guiding me closer to my soul's calling.

Challenges are an inevitable part of any journey. They come in various forms—external obstacles, internal struggles, and unexpected setbacks. But within each challenge lies a potential lesson, an opportunity to heal something within that wants to be healed, a chance to grow stronger and more self-aware.

Embracing these challenges is part of discovering your amazing authentic power.

During my time with the Maasai, I faced physical challenges, from adapting to a new environment to overcoming illness. Yet, the greatest challenges were internal. I had to confront my preconceived notions and biases, learning to see the world through different eyes. It was a humbling experience, teaching me the value of humility and the importance of staying open to new perspectives. Each challenge, rather than being a barrier, became a stepping stone in my journey toward greater self-awareness and empowerment.

Clarity often comes in the quiet moments of reflection that follow intense experiences. It's the moment when the noise subsides, and you can see the bigger picture, understanding the lessons learned. This clarity is essential for healing and empowerment because it allows you to align with your true purpose.

For me, clarity came in moments of solitude, away from the hustle and bustle of daily life. It was in the stillness of the Kenyan savannah or the tranquil Amazon rainforest that I could hear the whispers of my soul, guiding me toward my true path. These moments of clarity were transformative, providing me with a deeper understanding of who I am and what I'm meant to do in this world.

It was through a near death experience that I discovered my soul's purpose. I was traveling in Uganda and went to Bwindi Park to see the mountain gorillas. It was one of the most amazing experiences of my life, hiking through the jungle for a few hours and then sitting near a family of gorillas, watching them interact. On the way down, the brakes failed on the SUV I was in. The emergency brake didn't work either. Instead of going over the 1000 ft cliff, the driver hit the side of the mountain at high speed, and the vehicle flew up in the air and rolled four times, landing on the roof. Sliding down that dirt road upside down, I knew we were heading to the cliff and was certain we would die. I felt the fear of death and silently prayed over and over, "God, please save us." The windows had blown out, and the vehicle was caving in on us. Finally, just 3 feet before the edge of the cliff, the vehicle stopped. We survived. As banged up as I was, I knew I was meant to live and that I had something important to do. That new inner knowing changed the course of my life.

Interestingly enough, my best friend, who often told me I was a healer, had insisted on me taking a huge book on various healing modalities with me to Africa. I resisted as it was a large book and took up so much space in my backpack, but I finally agreed. The trip down off that mountain and back to my hut was grueling, but I pulled that book out and started trying out the various energy healing modalities. I healed myself of the PTSD I suffered after that accident. I finally accepted that I was a healer. Once back home, I immediately registered for a diploma program in acupressure and continued training in various modalities and healing others.

I learned that the near-fatal accident was what it took for me to accept my soul's purpose. I realized that the Universe had been speaking through my friend all those years, and I was the one getting in my own way from becoming the energy healer and teacher I was born to be.

Every journey has a return, a moment when you come back to your starting point but as a changed person. You return with newfound wisdom, insights, and a deeper sense of self. This return is not just about coming back physically but about integrating the healing and empowerment you experienced into your everyday life.

When I returned from my travels, I was no longer the same person who had set out. I had done a lot of deep healing along the way, gained a wealth of experiences and insights that enriched my life and my work. I brought back with me a deeper appreciation for diversity, a stronger sense of purpose, and a renewed commitment to helping others on their own journeys of healing and empowerment. The journey had transformed me, enabling me to live life as a much greater and authentic version of myself.

Ultimately, the journey of healing and empowerment leads you to live your soul's purpose. It's about discovering who you truly are and aligning your life with your deepest values and passions. This journey is not a one-time event but a continual process of growth and discovery. Living your soul's purpose means embracing your unique gifts and using them to make a positive impact in the world. It's about appreciating the lessons learned, opening up to deep healing, and moving into your authentic power while remaining open to the endless possibilities that lie ahead. My journey taught me that true empowerment comes from within, from the courage to be yourself and the willingness to embark on your own journey, no matter how challenging it may seem.

Healing and empowerment are indeed a profound exploration, a journey that takes you well beyond your comfort zone and into the realms of self-discovery and transformation. By courageously embracing this journey, you open yourself up to a world of possibilities, unlocking the potential within you to live a life of purpose and fulfillment. As you continue on this path, remember that every step you take brings you closer to your truest self and the incredible life you are destined to live.

Is it necessary to sell everything and travel in developing countries? Absolutely not. That was part of my journey. Where are you on your journey? You have likely picked up this book because you know something needs to change. Is it a relationship? Or is it your career or business? Do you have an inner knowing that you must do something about your health? It might even be that you feel the call to grow spiritually.

Before we move on, I'd like to share a story of Sam, who found my book, Heal Your Neck Issues and Let Your Throat Chakra Shine. She read the book and near the end of our discovery call, said, "Well, I want to work with you because I know the meditations work. I've done them. I want to work on healing myself so I can step into who I truly am. It's just a matter of how much it costs." Sam had been working in the corporate world for years. She knew she had throat chakra issues and felt blocked around moving forward. She was serious about wanting clarity and change, and she got more clarity and change than she could have imagined.

"I was very conflicted in my life prior to working with Cheryl. And I felt that I couldn't communicate well, I felt that I was conflicted in my material world. And in my spiritual life, I felt like I was becoming more spiritual, and wasn't really sure where everything fitted into place. I was working a sort of corporate IT job, but felt like I needed something more and something was missing. I don't have that conflict anymore. I feel that I know where I want to be now in my spiritual world. I have discovered my love for plants and herbal healing, and really realized that I want to be a spiritual healer. And I can see myself transitioning now from that IT material world. I am so really positive, that I can move forward. I don't have so much impostor syndrome anymore. I really believe in myself and have confidence. I think I was definitely in the need of some sort of spiritual mentoring and coaching somehow the Universe put me in touch with you. You know, I feel like I've really turned the corner that I needed to turn. I would certainly encourage anybody and say, Just do it. It's worth it. It'll get you where you need to be." - Sam Gordon

As you come to the close of this chapter, take a moment to reflect on your own journey. Healing and empowerment are more than just concepts; they are the keys to unlocking your true purpose and stepping into your authentic power. This journey is not always easy, but it is transformative. Each challenge you face, each block you clear, brings you closer to becoming the person you were always meant to be.

The stories shared here—whether they are of deep personal healing, the courage to step into the unknown, or the determination to live authentically—are reminders that the journey to your true purpose and authentic power is uniquely yours. It doesn't require you to sell everything or travel the world, but it does require you to listen to the call within, to be brave enough to explore the depths of your being, and to embrace the process of transformation.

Remember, the privilege of a lifetime is to become who you truly are, who and what your soul came here to be. As you continue on this path, know that every step, every moment of clarity, and every bit of healing brings you closer to living your soul's purpose and embodying your authentic power which is, ultimately, divine power moving through you. Trust in the journey, and allow yourself to step fully into the empowered, authentic life you are destined to live.

13

Spike of Purpose

"Purpose is the reason you journey. Passion is the fire that lights your way." — *Anonymous*

In a world full of opportunities and distractions, many women feel a longing for a deeper sense of purpose. Despite their achievements and personal growth, there's often an inner voice whispering that they are meant for more. This chapter aims to guide you, a woman who has already done significant personal work, towards discovering and embracing your true purpose. (Works for men also.)

Purpose is not just about what you do; it's about who you are at your core. It's the unique expression of your soul's calling, the reason you wake up each morning with excitement and fulfillment. It goes beyond job titles, societal expectations, and material achievements. Purpose is the inner fire that fuels your passion, your drive, and your ability to impact the world meaningfully.

My journey toward discovering my purpose was profoundly shaped by a near-death experience in Uganda. During that harrowing moment, I faced the reality of my own mortality. In the midst of fear and uncertainty, a deep, inner knowing emerged—an understanding that my life was spared because I still had something important to accomplish. This realization became a turning point, infusing my life with a renewed sense of purpose and direction. This experience taught me that life is precious and that each of us has a unique mission to fulfill. What I didn't see at that time was that my purpose was right in front of me. It was inside me. I was living and breathing my purpose; I just needed to acknowledge it, accept it, and allow it.

A couple of years after that experience, I did a week-long personal meditation retreat by myself in my home. I was in a spiritual school at the time that had retreat guides. The president of the school contacted me when she found out I was going to do this without a guide. I let her know I had done vision quests and personal retreats by myself, with and without a guide, and that I was looking forward to it. She had never done this herself, so I understood her concern and convinced her I would be fine. It was at the end of my seven days of meditating for hours at a time when it came to me suddenly, like a lightning bolt out of the sky. It was the unmistakable guidance I heard that will ring in my ears forever: "You are a spiritual teacher." I burst into tears and wept. I could feel the profound truth in this guidance, yet it felt like it was too much for me to acknowledge and fully accept, let alone step into. Sure, I was already a meditation teacher and helped a lot of people in many ways, but it was always part-time.

Five months later, I did another retreat and was guided by that teacher in person. At the end of that retreat, I received the same message. This time I could acknowledge and accept it. She reminded me that the first time she met me, she gave me that same guidance during a Darshan. I had forgotten about it, but once mentioned, I remembered thinking she was crazy and didn't know what she was talking about. Here I was a year later, sitting with acceptance and knowing that would form my future but not knowing what it would look like. Things started to fall into place, and my spiritual business grew and grew into a thriving and deeply fulfilling enterprise. I continue to grow and evolve through my business. I often say:

> *"Whenever you take a giant step forward, whatever kept you from doing that before will come up."*
>
> — *Cheryl Stelte*

The challenges keep coming, and the healing and empowerment become easier, or at least more familiar. It's a choice to engage fully with life and the Universe at this level. The rewards are immeasurable.

Embracing your purpose is a journey, not a destination. It requires courage, trust, and a willingness to step out of your comfort zone. As you begin to uncover your purpose, you may face fears and doubts. These are natural parts of the process and indicators that you are on the right path. To fully embrace your purpose, surround yourself with a supportive community. Seek out mentors, friends, and groups that resonate with your values and aspirations. Share your journey with them and allow their encouragement to bolster your confidence.

Living your purpose means aligning your daily actions with your deepest values and passions. It's about being authentic, courageous, and compassionate. When you live from a place of purpose, you inspire others to do the same. Your life becomes a testament to the power of clarity, healing, and empowerment. You can do all the traditional things: set intentions, create vision boards, set achievable goals, and celebrate your progress. The key is to imagine how it feels to be living a life of purpose. Imagine the emotions you will experience when your life is fulfilling. That, to me, is what you want to return to. Do whatever makes you feel that way. I spent my time traveling searching for purpose when it was right inside me. My travels were a spiritual pilgrimage. I loved to do anything spiritual that helped me grow and evolve and had been that way for years. Remember, your purpose is not a rigid path but a dynamic, evolving journey. Embrace the twists and turns with whatever grace you can muster and trust that you are exactly where you need to be.

Discovering your true purpose is a profound and transformative journey. It requires getting out of your own way and not trying too hard. It is not to be found outside you but within you. It requires the courage to step into your highest potential. As you embrace a sense of purpose, you will not only find fulfillment and joy but also become a beacon of light and inspiration for others. You are meant for more. You are here to make a difference. Let the sense of purpose and the emotions that go with it be your guiding star, illuminating your path and empowering you to create a life beyond what you have ever dreamed of. I never imagined or dreamed of doing what I do. Remember, you are powerful beyond belief, powerful beyond what you can imagine.

The day I discovered the spike of purpose during a chakra reading is still vivid in my mind. It was a transformative moment while working with an older woman, whom I'll call Jane. At the beginning of the session, I asked Jane about her intentions and silently invoked spiritual guidance through prayer. Once I relayed the message I received for Jane from the Universe, my focus turned to her root chakra. As I shared my observations, a peculiar sight caught my attention—a long, cone-shaped band of light energy extending behind her root chakra. Intrigued by this unfamiliar phenomenon, I ventured further, guided by curiosity and intuition. What I uncovered within Jane was profound—a resolute sense of purpose emanating from this cone-shaped band of light. It seemed as though Jane possessed a clear understanding of her life's purpose, a clarity that resonated deeply within her being. When I shared this insight with Jane, she acknowledged its truth, yet expressed a sense of untapped potential, an acknowledgment that there was more to explore and uncover within herself.

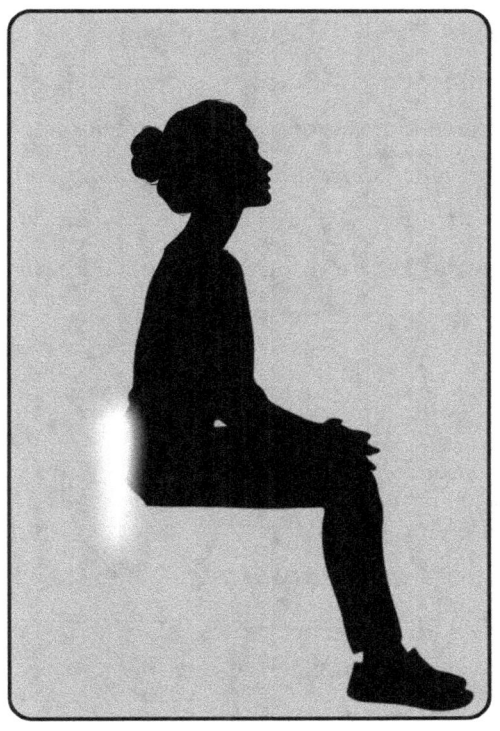

I call this energy the Spike of Purpose because it provides a stable foundation, connecting us to the Earth. It's like a vertical tent spike that anchors you firmly; no matter how strong the winds blow, it keeps you grounded and secure. You can always lean back on it. This revelation marked the beginning of a transformative journey for me. Subsequently, I began to discern similar energies in many individuals during chakra readings. There was a noticeable discrepancy between younger adults and older individuals who had accrued life experience. While the former often lacked the depth and clarity of purpose, the latter exhibited varying qualities within their spike of purpose. Those who had found fulfillment in their careers or personal lives radiated with bright, vibrant energy, while others who felt dissatisfied or unfulfilled emanated dark, brittle energy, or no energy at all. This distinctive pattern manifested as a long, narrow cone of varying sizes and brightness, each conveying a unique story of purpose and potential.

Recognizing the significance of this discovery, I made a conscious decision to integrate the analysis of the spike of purpose into all my chakra readings. I found it to be a powerful tool for self-awareness and personal growth, not only for my clients but also for myself. I encouraged each individual to explore this energy within themselves, to recognize their inherent potential, and to embrace the simplicity of breathing into their spike of purpose. Aligning intentions with purpose became a central focus, allowing energy to flow effortlessly and harmoniously.

Spike of Purpose Meditation

> ➢ *Begin: Sitting up very straight, with your feet on the floor, I invite you to get into your body and set your intention for this meditation. Begin with the Full Breath.*
> ➢ *Focus your awareness on the tip of your tailbone: And then let your inner gaze extend slightly behind it. Envision the spike of purpose descending along the coccyx, and breathe into that area. Then*

you can begin to mentally affirm the word "purpose."
- *Visualize Your Spike of Purpose and Breath Into It With a Full Breath: Picture your spike of purpose clearly in your mind. See its color, shape, and brightness. Observe how it changes and evolves as you focus on it.*
- *Tune into Sensations: Pay attention to any physical sensations you experience. Notice how your body feels in response to focusing on your spike of purpose. Breathe into the physical sensation while keeping your focus on the Spike of Purpose. What are the emotions held in the sensations? What wants to be felt?*
- *Use the ACE Method, provided earlier in this book. Access, Clear and Empower. By releasing subconscious barriers, you pave the way for realizing your purpose, beyond what you can currently imagine.*
- *Uncover Emotions in Memories: Allow any relevant memories or experiences to surface. This is an opportunity to cultivate curiosity and embrace both the joys and challenges inherent in pursuing your purpose. As you breathe deeply, let any memories or experiences float to the surface. Don't overthink them—just use the full depth of your breath to explore the feelings connected to these memories. Instead of trying to analyze with your*

mind, let your breath guide you into the emotions of these experiences. Dive into how you felt in those moments. Allow your breath to lead you deeper into your subconscious, unlocking insights about your true self. You might want to journal about these memories later, but for now, stay with the emotions. Let the memories unfold and see where the feelings take you. Notice how these memories or experiences relate to your current life. This is a time to be curious and open, to understand how both the good and tough times have shaped who you are. Use this moment to connect more deeply with yourself, guided by your breath and feelings.

- Ask Probing Questions: Once you have moved through any emotional barriers. While breathing deeply and keeping your focus on your spike of purpose, consider asking yourself these questions. Stay engaged with your intuitive, right brain rather than the analytical, left brain. Breathe fully and let your body, the part connected to the Spike of Purpose, respond. Wait for the answers to emerge from this inner connection.
- What is my soul responsible for?
- What is mine to accomplish?
- When I'm on my deathbed, what will I be grateful I accomplished?

> *What is the next step in my soul's journey?*
> *How have my life challenges contributed to my personal growth?*
> *What lessons have I learned through overcoming adversity?*
> *How can I use my experiences to fulfill my purpose?*
> *Reflect on how these questions apply to your current life situation. Allow the answers to emerge naturally, guiding you toward a deeper understanding of your purpose.*

When you view your life from a broader perspective and open your inner eyes to recognize that ALL your challenges have served you, facilitating growth in various aspects. I often emphasize that only the old souls willingly undertake experiences with the most profound difficulties and adversity. Yet, it is within these challenges that these old souls, acknowledging their inherent resilience (which exists within us all), find opportunities for profound growth. Each challenge we encounter serves as a catalyst for our evolution towards purpose.

Allowance and acceptance are crucial in this journey of self-discovery. Your higher self, with its profound understanding, can guide you beyond the shallow perceptions and limited beliefs of your smaller self. By cultivating a sense of allowance and acceptance, you can transcend the limitations of your ego and connect with the deeper wisdom of your soul.

Unlocking your Soul's Calling involves embracing responsibility and surrendering to the wisdom of your Spike of purpose. It is a journey of trust, faith, and responsibility, allowing you to align with your soul's purpose and embark on a path of fulfillment and self-realization. In surrender lies the key to unlocking the full potential of your Spike of purpose, allowing you to connect with the profound knowing within and letting your purpose unfold organically.

By expanding upon these concepts and delving deeper into the exploration of purpose, you can enrich your understanding and experience of the Spike of purpose within yourself. Through continued practice and reflection, you can align with your soul's calling and embark on a journey of profound growth and fulfillment. You can unlock the full potential of your Spike of purpose and step into the true essence of who you are.

Embracing your Soul's Calling requires a blend of trust, faith, and responsibility. Trust the inner guidance that arises within you, have faith in your capacity to fulfill your purpose, and take ownership of your journey. Aligning with your Soul's Calling allows your purpose to guide you toward a life rich in meaning and fulfillment, enabling you to fully embrace your true essence.

As you finish this chapter, keep in mind that your Spike of Purpose energetically grounds you, providing greater stability from your soul's knowing as you navigate life's challenges and opportunities. By trusting in your inner wisdom, having faith in your mission, and living authentically, you unlock your full potential. Let your purpose be the guiding light on your path to profound growth, fulfillment, and impact.

14

Clearing Blocks in Your Environment

"The space in which we live should be for the person we are becoming now, not for the person we were in the past."

— *Marie Kondo*

Have you ever walked into a room and felt an inexplicable sense of calm or, conversely, an uneasy feeling? Our environments profoundly affect our inner states, often in ways we might not consciously recognize. Through Denise Linn's training in Instinctive Feng Shui and Interior Alignment, I gained profound insights into how our surroundings can influence our mental and emotional well-being. By clearing blocks in our environment, we can pave the way to clear the blocks within ourselves, fostering a harmonious balance between our inner and outer worlds.

Instinctive Feng Shui is an intuitive approach to traditional Feng Shui principles. Unlike classical Feng Shui, which relies heavily on specific rules and compass directions, Instinctive Feng Shui emphasizes tuning into the natural energy flows of a space and making adjustments based on what feels right. This method encourages us to trust our instincts and create environments that resonate with our unique energy signatures.

Interior Alignment, another cornerstone of Denise Linn's training, is about aligning our living spaces with our personal energy to support our goals and aspirations. It involves not only clearing clutter but also arranging furniture, and using colors, textures, and elements so that energy flows well in the space. We also want to use items that reflect our true selves. The core idea is that our homes should be sanctuaries that nurture and inspire us. I had the privilege of studying with Denise Linn over 25 years ago, and her teachings have profoundly shaped my approach to creating harmonious environments for my clients and myself personally.

As you embark on the journey of clearing your environment, it's essential to ask your body for guidance and trust your intuition. Your body is a sensitive instrument that can provide valuable insights into what changes are needed in your space.

These methods can be applied not only to your home but also to your office, career, or business. A cluttered and chaotic workspace can lead to scattered thoughts and decreased productivity, while a well-organized and harmonious office can enhance focus and creativity. By applying these principles in your professional environment, you can create a space that supports your career aspirations and business goals.

Living Space Attunement: Before making any adjustments, take a moment to sit up straight in a chair and center yourself. Close your eyes, relax your body, feeling your feet on the floor. Give yourself plenty of time to engage in the Full Breath and ask your body how it feels in different areas of your home. Pay attention to any sensations or emotions that arise. These feelings will guide you to the areas that need the most attention.

Clutter is more than just a physical mess; it can be a manifestation of mental and emotional blockages. When our spaces are cluttered, our minds often feel scattered and overwhelmed. The first step in clearing blocks in your environment is to declutter.

Begin by looking around the room you are currently in. What stands out to you as holding energy that is not in alignment with who you truly are? Go up to any piece and hold it to your heart chakra. If it's a piece of furniture, put your left hand on it and your right hand on your heart chakra. Inhale the energy of the piece. How does it feel?

When I do this exercise for anything, including supplements, if something holds negative energy, my eyebrows and even my entire face scrunch up. If it is in alignment with my true self, my eyebrows lift up and I experience light. I experience unharmonious energy, angry or strong buzzing for negative energy, and harmonious sounds and strong light if positive energy. Students of this practice need time to map their own indicating sensations.

As you sort through your belongings, ask yourself: Do I love this item? Does it still serve me? Does it bring me joy? Is it in alignment with who I truly am or who I am becoming? If the answer is no, it might be time to let it go. If it is yes, where would it like to be placed? Find a designated place for everything you choose to keep. An organized space can reduce stress and enhance your sense of being in the flow of life.

This principle extends to your office or workspace. A cluttered desk can lead to a cluttered mind, making it difficult to focus on tasks and think creatively. Clear your desk of unnecessary items, keep only what is essential, and organize your workspace to promote efficiency and productivity. Consider the flow of energy in your office—ensure that your desk is in a commanding position, which is with your back to a wall and facing a window or door, and that you have a clear view of the entrance. Personalize your workspace with items that inspire you and reflect your professional goals.

Once you have cleared the clutter, the next step is to harmonize your space. This involves arranging your home to support the free flow of energy ("chi") and align with your personal intentions. Position your furniture to promote a smooth flow of energy, avoiding blocked pathways. Ensure that main pieces, like your bed and sofa, are placed in commanding positions (facing the door but not directly in line with it). In Feng Shui, you would incorporate the five elements—wood, fire, earth, metal, and water—to balance your environment. I prefer to use the four elements from indigenous cultures—earth, water, fire, and air—to achieve this balance. Regardless of the method you choose, each element has specific qualities and can be represented through colors, shapes, and materials. Infuse your space with items that reflect the person you are destined to become and what you want to feel more of—your fully aligned, powerful self. Artwork, photographs, and meaningful objects can enhance the emotional and energetic resonance of your home.

In your office, the arrangement of furniture and the inclusion of elements can also play a significant role in fostering a productive and positive work environment. Ensure that your workspace allows for the free flow of energy, with clear pathways and an organized layout. Incorporate symbols and elements that resonate with your professional aspirations—use colors that stimulate creativity and focus, and include plants or natural elements to bring in grounding energy. The addition of personal touches, such as awards, certificates, or motivational quotes, can remind you of your achievements and goals.

While I like to make my entire home a sacred space, creating specific sacred spaces within your home that are dedicated to relaxation, reflection, and spiritual practices will naturally enhance your life. These spaces can help you connect more deeply with your inner self and foster a sense of peace and clarity. Select a location that feels peaceful and away from high-traffic areas. Your sacred space doesn't need to be elaborate. A peaceful room, a small altar, or a meditation chair can suffice. Include items that inspire you—crystals, candles, incense, or sacred texts. The goal is to create a space where you feel how you wish to feel. You will notice that if you meditate in the same spot every day, the energy of meditation stays and over time, when you return to that space you will slip into meditation more quickly and with greater ease.

Regularly clearing the energy in your home can help maintain a positive and vibrant environment. Here are some techniques inspired by Denise Linn's teachings: Use sage or other herbs to cleanse your space of stagnant or negative energy. I have used sage, sandalwood, cedar, and juniper to cleanse a space. You can light the smudge stick or use a fresh branch from a plant. If lit, allow the smoke to waft through each room, and set an intention for clearing and renewal. Use bells, singing bowls, or chimes to break up and disperse negative energy. And like everything else, please take some time to meditate on your space-clearing ally. For me, it is cymbals. Walk through your home, gently or loudly ringing the instrument and visualizing the sound waves purifying your space. Place bowls of salt or crystals like amethyst and clear quartz in various rooms to absorb negative energy and promote a balanced atmosphere.

Fire Ceremony

A fire ceremony is a powerful ritual for releasing old patterns, negativity, and blocks, and for inviting new intentions, clarity, and transformation. Denise did such a beautiful fire ceremony during our training, I was in tears at the end. I have since done fire ceremonies numerous times over the years. It is the most powerful and sacred method used to clear the energy in a home or office. I recommend doing the fire ceremony in the center of your home or office. I usually create an altar on the floor with a beautiful piece of fabric and meaningful objects with pure intentions.

To perform this ceremony indoors, you will need an oven-proof dish, isopropyl alcohol, Epsom salts, matches or a lighter, paper and pen, and a small bowl of water. Optional items include sage or incense for smudging. To prepare for your ceremony, I recommend having clean clothes made of natural fiber ready and having a shower, rubbing your body with salt to be in your purest form possible.

Begin by finding the center of your home, or if that doesn't work, choosing a quiet, safe place indoors where you can perform the ceremony without interruptions. Ideally, create a sacred altar in the center of your home, placing the oven-proof dish on the floor. Ensure proper ventilation and have your materials nearby. Start by creating a sacred space.

Next, sit quietly for a few moments to center yourself. Close your eyes, using the Full Breath, tune into your heart chakra, asking what wants to be released. Write down what you wish to release from your life, such as old habits, *negative thoughts, unproductive ways of doing business, or fears. When complete, repeat the process and ask what wants to be created. Again, write down your intentions or what you wish to invite into your life, such as clarity, new opportunities, healing, the next phase of your business, or other specific goals.*

If you feel called to, you can honor the four directions (North, South, East, West) and the elements (Earth, Air, Fire, Water) to invite their energies into your ceremony. Face each direction, acknowledge it, and invite its presence.

To prepare the fire, pour Epsom salts into the oven-proof dish and then pour isopropyl alcohol over the salts until they are saturated but not swimming. Place the dish on a trivet. Safely light the mixture in the dish. As the fire grows, focus on its transformative power. Read your intentions silently or out loud energetically exhale each intention into the fire. You can say something like, "I release these with love and gratitude."

Then, read your intentions regarding what you would like to invite in. As you do, say something like, "I invite these blessings into my life." Visualize the smoke carrying your intentions to the Universe. Spend a few moments in silence, expressing gratitude for the transformation and for the elements that assisted you in the ceremony.

Once you feel complete, thank the fire for its transformative power and safely extinguish it with the bowl of water if necessary. Ensure the fire is completely out before leaving the space. Finally, take a few deep breaths, and visualize any remaining energy grounding into the earth. You can also place your hands on the ground to help with grounding.

Reflect on the experience and any insights or feelings that arose during the ceremony. Consider journaling about the ceremony and any shifts you notice in the days and weeks following. Stay open to the new opportunities and changes that may come into your life as a result of the ceremony. Remember, a fire ceremony is a deeply personal ritual, so feel free to adapt these steps to suit your own needs and preferences. The most important aspect is your intention and presence during the process.

Clearing blocks in your environment supports clearing your internal blocks. As you clear physical clutter and obstacles, you will find it easier to address and remove internal blockages, and vice versa. To become a clear being of love and light, it helps to create a clear and loving space around you. Just like clearing your subconscious blocks, it is vital to reprogram your subconscious. The same applies to your home or environment. Objects are always giving us subliminal messages. By replacing old items that no longer serve you with specific items that are symbolic, lift you up, or help you feel powerful, the energy of those items will be reflected back to you. This reflection supports more reprogramming in your subconscious, enhancing your personal growth and inner clarity. As you surround yourself with objects that resonate with your true self, you strengthen the positive energy in your environment, which in turn nurtures your inner transformation. Often, when I receive an image of some type of significant symbolism in a healing and empowerment meditation, I either find a piece of art or most often, create a canvas print. I did that with the Statue of Liberty, which symbolizes freedom and enlightening the world, which have become ideals for me. Also, the Eiffel Tower lights up the city. We can all be the energetic light for our cities. I have a beautiful statue of Sekhmet on my desk, gifted to me by a beloved client, to remind me of my purpose as a powerful healer.

In your business environment, consider what symbolic items might inspire and motivate you. Whether it's a piece of art that represents your company's mission, a plant that brings a sense of growth and renewal, or an object that symbolizes your professional aspirations, these items can reinforce positive messages and support your business goals.

Over the years, I have helped numerous clients sell their homes by identifying and removing items that held negative energy, preventing the home from selling. One client, desperate to sell her home, sought my help. She was willing to alter furniture placement or even paint the entire exterior a different color, although it didn't need new paint. While I did make a few suggestions on furniture placement, one particular item drew my attention in a room: a huge, tall basket standing on the floor. I didn't want to open it myself without the owner present. When she entered the room, I asked her about it and what was inside. She said it was full of gifts from her alcoholic daughter and son-in-law, gifts she couldn't stand to look at, so she hid them in the basket. Like many people, she felt obligated to keep these "gifts." I suggested she get rid of them as soon as possible. She removed the basket and its contents with loving intention and forgiveness, and she received an offer on her home within days.

Another couple, for whom I had done my largest renovation and a lot of spiritual work with the wife, Susan, shared with me one day that their home in another province had been on the market for 18 months and still hadn't sold. They offered to fly me out there with them to see if I could help it sell. I suggested instead that I do a reading on it first to see what the problem was, and Susan happily agreed. However, Jim, her husband, was skeptical.

During the reading, I received various insights and saw a row of trees behind the house. I sensed anger and resentment held there. When I called to report my findings, Susan was out of town, so I asked Jim if he would prefer to wait for Susan or hear the results himself. He wanted to know. When I mentioned the row of trees, he informed me that there was no row of trees. I was puzzled. After further inquiry, I asked, "Has there ever been a row of trees at the back of the house?" He told me there used to be a row of trees, but the neighbor behind them had cut them all down. His wife had been very angry and sad about losing those trees and had never really gotten over it.

When Susan returned, I worked with her to help release everything around that situation. Exactly one week later, the house was sold to a young family.

Throughout the process of clearing and harmonizing your space, remember to trust your intuition. Your inner guidance is a powerful tool that can lead you to make the right decisions for your environment. If something feels off or out of place, trust that feeling and make adjustments accordingly. Your intuition can also help you identify areas that need more attention or specific objects that may be holding negative energy.

Clearing blocks in your environment is a powerful step towards clearing the blocks within yourself. By applying the principles of Instinctive Feng Shui and Interior Alignment, you can transform your living space into a sanctuary that supports your well-being and personal growth. Applying these principles to your office and business environment can enhance your professional life, leading to greater clarity, productivity, and success. Remember to ask your body for guidance and trust your intuition throughout this process. Your home is an extension of your inner world, and when you create harmony in your environment, you pave the way for greater clarity, peace, and empowerment in your life.

15

Evolving Through Heart-Centered Shamanism

"The earth has music for those who listen."
— *William Shakespeare*

One of the most powerful practices I've discovered on my spiritual journey is called merging. It's a deep shamanic technique where you blend your energy with another being, like an animal or a deity, to gain wisdom and healing. This practice is based on the belief that everything has a spirit, and by connecting with these spirits, we can learn more about ourselves and the Universe. One of my teachers, Claude Poncelet, a shaman from Belgium, emphasized only using practices that resonate with us and becoming our own teachers.

During a workshop with Claude, elephant came to me immediately in the opening ritual. I discovered the personal benefits of merging, as elephant taught me to slow down. This was crucial to me as someone who often rushed through life, especially while running my spiritual interior design business and at the same time, working to overcome adrenal fatigue. By merging and connecting with power animals, you learn more about yourself, the qualities developing in you, and your authentic power, as well as the power of the Universe flowing through you.

Merging is different from another shamanic practice called shapeshifting, where you lose your sense of self entirely and completely become the other. Claude was an expert at this, but admitted he did too much of it at one time and it affected his health. In merging, you keep your own identity while blending with the other being. This allows you to experience both yourself and the other being at the same time, connecting with their essence.

Merging with great goddesses, gods, saints, spiritual masters or angelic beings lifts us up to states we couldn't achieve on our own. We access not only their essence and their much higher vibration, but also the great power these beings contain. This practice can be just as life changing for you as it has been for me. Doing this practice will help you become your powerful self beyond what you can currently imagine. This is the foundational exercise I teach in the Azarias Energy Healing Certification Program. In order to become powerful healers, we merge with Archangel Raphael and other beings. We open up to these great beings, becoming filled with light and love in order to allow them to heal through us. If we stop merging, we then return to our mortal selves and cannot help our client to release their energetic blocks.

Whenever I do chakra readings, I am always merging. I wouldn't be where I am today without merging. I can say I am a powerful healer only because I have developed a great capacity to allow the power of other beings to heal through me. I could share 100 stories here, but I would rather invite you to jump in and give it a try for yourself.

Practicing Merging: A Step-by-Step Guide

Find a quiet place to sit comfortably. Close your eyes, take deep breaths, and relax. Set a clear intention for the merge—whatever you hope to learn or achieve. This helps to focus your mind and will guide your experience. Use slow, Full Breaths to enter a calm, meditative state that's ideal for merging.

Visualize the being you want to merge with—whether a deity, person, or object. Remember, everything has a spirit. Open yourself up and then feel their spirit merging with yours as you breathe in their essence and expand your energy to connect with theirs. As you merge, open up to see things from their perspective and feel how they move or function in the world. This raises your awareness to discover more about yourself as well as aligning you with the Universe's energy.

Fully immerse yourself in the experience. Notice any sensations, emotions, or insights that arise. These may offer guidance, clarity, or healing as you align your energies with the being you've chosen. When you're ready to finish, thank the being or object for sharing their energy with you. Slowly return to your normal awareness, by taking a few deep breaths to ground yourself. Reflect on the merge's impact on you and on any new understandings you've gained.

Merging is a powerful tool for releasing emotional, mental, and energetic obstacles that hold you back. By connecting with another entity, you become more aware of internal barriers, making it easier to acknowledge, process, and let go of them. Merging isn't limited to animals; you can merge with plants, trees, crystals, or mountains. I spoke with a shaman once who told me she had the greatest insight ever when merging with a garbage dumpster. Every being and every thing offers unique teachings and perspectives. Plants share healing wisdom and a connection with nature. Trees symbolize strength and spiritual grounding. Crystals amplify energy and provide clarity. Mountains offer perspective and endurance in facing life's challenges. Other humans allow us the opportunity for greater compassion and understanding of another person.

Reflect on your merging experiences by journaling. Note any sensations, insights, or shifts in your emotions. Apply these insights to personal growth and decision-making, integrating the qualities of merged beings into your being and daily actions. Sharing your experiences with others builds community and deepens your understanding of spiritual guidance. By incorporating merging into your spiritual practice, life or business, you can clear blocks, gain clarity, and connect more deeply with the world around you and yourself.

Power Animals and Power Animal Retrieval

In shamanism, power animals are spiritual guides that offer wisdom, protection, and strength. Each power animal has unique qualities and abilities that can help guide you on our spiritual journey. These animals represent real energies and allies in the spiritual world, not just symbols.

In many tribal cultures around the world, people believed that every person was born with a power animal to support them on their journey. These power animals were seen as spiritual allies, offering guidance, protection, and strength throughout a person's life. They were an important part of the community's spiritual practices, connecting individuals with the natural world and the wisdom of the animal kingdom. Each power animal had unique qualities and lessons, perfectly matched to the person's life path and challenges. This deep bond with power animals created a harmonious relationship between humans and nature, grounding spiritual beliefs in the community's everyday experiences.

However, as people evolved and Westerners intruded, this sacred connection was often lost. The imposition of Western values and the disruption of traditional ways of life led to a disconnection from the natural world and the spiritual practices that sustained these communities. The loss of the power animal connection mirrored the broader erosion of indigenous cultures and their deep, intuitive understanding of the world. Today, there is a growing recognition of the importance of reconnecting with these ancient practices. By re-establishing our bond with power animals, we can reclaim a sense of balance, wisdom, and spiritual support that has been missing from our lives, enriching our personal journeys and deepening our connection to the natural world.

Power animals act as guides by sharing their special traits and strengths. For example, the eagle represents vision and a higher perspective, while the bear symbolizes strength and courage. By connecting with a power animal, you can use their wisdom and qualities to help you in your own life. Power animals serve as protectors and companions. They offer guidance, helping you understand your purpose and navigate difficult situations. They also provide energy and strength, empowering you to overcome obstacles and achieve your goals. Power animals often reflect parts of our personality or current life situations, making their guidance relevant and meaningful.

To find your power animal, you need to open up to receiving the spirit that will currently benefit you the most for where you are at. You can discover your birth power animal or a power animal that would benefit you in your life right now through shamanic journeying. Shamanic journeying helps you connect with the spiritual world and invite your power animal to reveal itself. Initially, I learned that shamanic journeying involved entering a trance state through the beat of the drum which represented the heartbeat of the earth, to connect with the spiritual world. Using rhythmic drumming or rattling, you can journey to a spiritual realm to meet your power animal. This often gives you a direct and powerful experience of your power animal's energy and guidance. However, after practicing these types of journeys and leaving my body to go to the lower world and upper world, I discovered that leaving the body is not necessary and also not healthy. I found it much safer and more effective to journey into one's heart chakra while staying fully present in our bodies.

Leaving the body during shamanic journeying can be risky and potentially unhealthy because it disrupts our connection to the present moment and our physical selves. When we leave our bodies, we may often become detached from the grounding and stabilizing influence of our physical form, leading to feelings of disorientation and dissociation. This detachment can make it difficult to process and integrate the insights and experiences gained during the journey. Additionally, it may expose us to negative energies or entities in the spiritual realm without the protective anchoring of our physical presence. Staying embodied during shamanic practices ensures that we remain connected to our natural state of being, allowing for a more balanced and harmonious integration of spiritual experiences into our everyday lives. This grounded approach promotes a healthier and more sustainable path of spiritual growth and healing.

The heart chakra is a powerful energy center that connects you to your emotions, love, and compassion. It is actually the most powerful chakra and the energetic hub of all the chakras. I have discovered that at the back bottom of the heart chakra is a special shamanic portal used for power animal retrieval. By accessing this portal, you can journey into a sacred space where your power animal will come to you. You can try this for yourself. Here's how:

Power Animal Retrieval Practise

Preparing for the Retrieval: *Start by finding a quiet place to meditate without interruptions. Sit comfortably and take several deep, Full Breaths. Focus on your heart chakra, located in the center of your chest and on the inside of your spine and imagine you are breathing there. Visualize a portal at the back bottom of your heart chakra, a glowing entrance to a sacred space within you.*

Entering the Sacred Space: *Continue breathing deeply and let your breath guide you into this portal. With each inhale, imagine yourself moving deeper into the space. Pay attention to how the space feels, looks, and smells. Notice the colors, textures, and any sensations that arise. This sacred space is where your power animal will reveal itself.*

Meeting Your Power Animal: *Once you are fully immersed in the space, invite your power animal to come forward. Be patient and open, allowing the animal to appear in its own time. Your power animal should come to you four times during the same meditation to confirm its identity. This repetition ensures that you recognize and connect with your true power animal. Observe their form, behavior, and* *energy as your power animal appears. Notice any feelings or messages they convey. Trust your intuition and the impressions you receive. The four encounters help you build a strong connection with your power animal, confirming their presence and guidance in your life.*

Returning and Integrating: *When ready to end the session, thank your power animal and slowly return to regular awareness. Visualize the portal at the back bottom of your heart chakra gently closing, sealing the sacred space. Take a few deep breaths and ground yourself by becoming aware of your surroundings. Reflect on your experience by journaling your insights and feelings. Note the characteristics of your power animal and any messages they conveyed to you. This will help you integrate the wisdom and guidance received during the retrieval.*

Connecting with your power animal offers many benefits. They provide guidance, helping you make decisions and understand your life's path. Their wisdom can offer new perspectives on challenges, leading to clearer solutions and profound insights. Power animals also offer protection and strength. Their energy can help you face fears and overcome obstacles, empowering you to navigate difficult situations with confidence. By embodying the qualities of your power animal, you can tap into their courage, resilience, and wisdom. Additionally, power animals enhance your spiritual connection. They serve as intermediaries between you and the spiritual world, helping you deepen your relationship with the divine. This connection fosters a sense of unity with nature and the spiritual realm, enriching your spiritual practice and personal growth.

Building a strong relationship with your power animal involves regular communication and honoring their presence in your life. Start by acknowledging and respecting your power animal's energy. You can do this through meditation, offerings, or simply expressing gratitude. Regular meditation or journeying sessions with your power animal can strengthen your bond. During these sessions, invite your power animal to share their wisdom and guidance. Ask questions about your life, challenges, or spiritual growth, and trust the insights they offer. Honoring your power animal can also involve integrating their qualities into your daily life. Reflect on how you can embody their strengths, such as courage, patience, or creativity. By living in alignment with your power animal's traits, you deepen your connection and make their energy a part of your everyday experience.

Power animals are vital allies in shamanic practice, offering wisdom, protection, and strength. By connecting with your power animal through the heart chakra, you can gain valuable guidance and support for your spiritual journey. Identifying your power animal involves recognizing the spirit that resonates with your essence, while power animal retrieval through the heart chakra provides a unique method for restoring lost connections and renewing your spiritual energy. This connection enhances your spiritual growth, empowers you to overcome challenges, and deepens your relationship with the natural and spiritual worlds. Embrace the journey of discovering and connecting with your power animal. Their presence can guide you toward greater clarity, strength, and spiritual fulfillment, supporting you on your path to personal and spiritual growth and empowerment.

As you close this chapter, remember that evolving through heart-centered shamanism is a journey of deep connection, self-discovery, and empowerment. By engaging in practices like merging and power animal retrieval, you open yourself to the wisdom and guidance of the spiritual world, enriching your life in profound ways. I encourage you to embrace these ancient tools with an open heart, and allow them to guide you toward a life of greater clarity, strength, and spiritual fulfillment. Through these sacred connections, you can access more of the authentic power within and around you, stepping more fully into the person you are meant to be.

16

Take Your Seat

"The future belongs to those who believe in the beauty of their dreams."

— *Eleanor Roosevelt*

This chapter is about embracing your soul's mission and stepping into your power. You are destined for greatness! The concept of taking your seat is more than just a metaphor; it's about claiming your rightful place in the world and embodying your true potential. When you start this process, you do not need to have any idea whatsoever of your purpose.

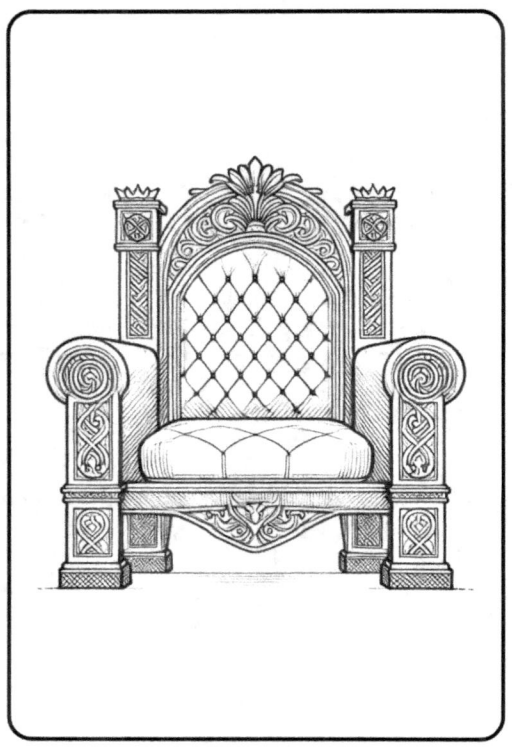

Imagine there is a gorgeous, lavish, golden throne right in front of you. This is your throne and you feel it is calling you to take your seat and own your place. This throne represents your innate wisdom, strength, and authority. It's a place where you connect deeply with your soul's purpose and confidently navigate life's challenges and opportunities to fulfill your soul's purpose.

Stepping into your greatness means acknowledging your unique gifts and strengths. It's about cultivating a deep trust in yourself and in the Universe, transcending mere safety and stability to embrace growth and expansion.

I remember a pivotal meditation years ago where suddenly, a large, beautiful, ornate golden throne appeared before me. It was a powerful symbol of empowerment and clarity. It was such a profound experience for me and it felt like the whole universe wanted me to take my seat, to own my destiny, and live from this place of empowerment. Unfortunately, at that time, my insecurities resurfaced. I felt unready, not good enough, and unworthy. Unbeknownst to me, I had a deep-seated fear of embracing my authentic power, not fully understanding that the highest level of my authentic power involves opening up to allowing divine power to flow through me. So, I passed on the opportunity. This was the second time I had turned down a significant spiritual opportunity for growth and stepping into my true power. Reflecting on these experiences, I later realized that my soul had chosen to face deep wounds and traumas related to feelings of inadequacy and unworthiness. Over time, I healed these wounds as much as I could and embraced "taking my seat" and also owning my purpose in the world.

A throne is more than just an ornate chair; it symbolizes power, authority, and sovereignty. Throughout history and across cultures, thrones have served as potent symbols of leadership and rulership. Sitting upon a throne signifies the culmination of personal and spiritual growth, where one embraces their true essence and steps into a position of influence. It represents a place of honor and dignity, where decisions are made and responsibilities accepted.

The symbolism of the throne extends beyond mere physicality; it embodies spiritual significance as well. In many spiritual traditions, the throne is seen as a sacred seat of divine authority or enlightenment. It signifies a connection to higher realms of consciousness and spiritual wisdom.

Moreover, sitting on a throne implies a balance between power and humility. It's not just about exerting authority, it's more about serving others with wisdom and compassion. A true leader on their throne listens to their people, understands their needs, and leads with integrity. It's harder to run away from life's problems if you are sitting on a throne.

In personal development, the concept of the throne can be metaphorical—a representation of inner strength, self-awareness, and clarity. It symbolizes the journey towards self-mastery and the realization of one's potential. This is about you living your soul's purpose, stepping into your greatness, and making a meaningful impact in the world.

Let's further explore what it means to "take your seat" on your metaphorical throne and how you can embody the qualities of a leader in your own life, embracing your innate power and purpose. By understanding the symbolism of the throne, you will learn to navigate challenges with grace and lead with authenticity, fulfilling your destiny with confidence.

The queen or king archetype embodies sovereignty, power, and leadership, transcending mere authority to encompass a deep sense of responsibility and wisdom. As an archetype, it symbolizes the pinnacle of personal and spiritual development, where one has integrated the lessons of the lower chakras—root, sacral, solar plexus, and heart—into a cohesive whole. Like a monarch, the queen or king archetype represents balance: the ability to receive and express, to delegate and decide with clarity and confidence. It signifies a state of inner knowing and strength, where one sits in their metaphorical throne not only as a leader in their own life but also as a beacon of guidance and inspiration for others on their journeys of growth and self-discovery.

In your journey of discovering your personal power, taking your seat means acknowledging your unique gifts and strengths. It's about cultivating a deep trust in yourself and in the Universe, transcending mere safety and stability to embrace growth and expansion. This is about aligning with who you truly are and making a meaningful impact in the world. A meaningful impact in the world can be through your business, career, volunteering, motherhood or grandmotherhood, creating community, being a silent leader, finding ways to express love, saving the rainforest, finding opportunities to be kind and compassionate, or a million other ways. It's about allowing your specific way or ways to come to you.

I often think of Queen Elizabeth, whose father passed when she was a mere 18 years of age. She ascended to the throne amidst profound grief and tremendous uncertainty. Yet, she embraced her role with a steadfast determination that mirrored the strength of her ancestors. In her coronation speech, she pledged her life to the service of her people, embodying the essence of duty, grace, and resilience. Throughout her reign, she navigated turbulent times with unwavering composure, earning the admiration and respect of her nation and the world. Her ability to unite, to lead with humility and wisdom, continues to inspire generations, reminding us that true leadership transcends individual challenges to leave a lasting legacy of courage and dedication.

Taking your seat involves owning your decisions and responsibilities, even amidst uncertainties. You don't have to know entirely what you are doing, you just need to own your place in the world and it will all come to you.

For now, I encourage you to practice the meditation at the end of this chapter until it feels natural, even uplifting and joyful. Pay attention to any uncomfortable emotions that surface. This is one of the practices in this book that is designed to help you surrender to the unknown, to surrender to your own innate inner power, which is currently hidden inside you.

In many self-help books and coaching programs, the typical approach involves setting clear goals, crafting a vision for the future, and engaging in analytical thinking. Questions like "What is my true calling?" and "Where can I make a meaningful impact?" are often used to guide this process. However, my approach here diverges from this traditional path. Instead of relying solely on the analytical left brain, which you may have already explored extensively, let me emphasize that tapping into the intuitive and creative right brain is where all the action is.

The essence of finding clarity and uncovering your soul's purpose lies in creating ample space within your right brain to receive insights and guidance. Unlike the logical left brain, which focuses on structure and analysis, the right brain excels in creativity, intuition, and holistic thinking. It allows us to access deeper layers of understanding and connect with our inner wisdom that often eludes us in the busyness of everyday life.

I firmly believe, because of my experience, that within each of us lies the potential to discover profound truths and insights about our life's purpose. By quieting the analytical mind and opening up to the intuitive channels of the right brain, you can begin to sense and understand your soul's calling more clearly. This journey isn't about forcing answers or setting rigid goals; it's about creating a receptive state where clarity naturally emerges from within.

For now, please just trust the process. Practice this meditation at least six times and journal about how it felt, noting all your uncomfortable and uplifting emotions.

The meditation practice provided here serves as a gateway to a receptive state. As you engage with it, allow yourself to relax and be present with whatever physical sensations and/or emotions arise. This practice isn't just about relaxation; it's about surrendering to the unknown and embracing the innate power that resides within you, that may be hidden beneath layers of everyday concerns, distractions, wounds, and traumas. Through this process of surrender and self-discovery, you can gradually unveil your true purpose and align more deeply with the path that brings you fulfillment and joy.

Engage with the meditation practice provided and allow yourself the time and space to embody this meditation in all your cells, in your entire being, knowing that clarity unfolds through the act of claiming your sovereignty. This ongoing practice of taking your seat is a journey toward personal and spiritual growth—a commitment to actualizing your greatness and embracing the responsibilities that come with it.

As we embark on this path together, remember that From Blocked To Powerful is not just about achieving external success; it's about aligning with your soul's purpose and making a meaningful impact. By embracing your inner sovereign and stepping into your power, you unlock the limitless potential within you and pave the way for profound transformations.

Meditation: Take Your Seat

Part 1: Root Chakra Activation

> - Begin by finding a comfortable seated position in a chair with your spine straight and feet flat on the floor. Close your eyes and take a few deep belly breaths, inhaling to 6-8 seconds slowly through your nose and exhaling gently for 6-8 seconds through your nose. Let your body relax with each breath.

> *Bring your attention to your root chakra, located at the tip of your tailbone. As you focus on this area, imagine a warm, glowing light gathering there. This light represents the energy of your root chakra.*
> *Breathe deeply into your root chakra. As you inhale, silently say to yourself the words "love" and "light." Feel these words filling your root chakra with warmth and energy. As you exhale, let go of any tension or negativity, allowing your body to relax even more.*
> *Focus on developing safety and stability. Imagine this light in your root chakra growing stronger, creating a foundation of safety and stability. Allow yourself to feel grounded, secure, and supported by this energy. If you feel unsafe or unstable, take your time to strengthen this foundation before moving on.*

Part 2: Trust and Faith

> *Once you feel a strong sense of safety and stability, begin to breathe into the words "trust" and "faith." Imagine these words blending with the light in your root chakra, enhancing your connection to yourself and the Universe.*
> *Allow yourself to trust in your journey. Feel a sense of faith in your ability to navigate life and its challenges. Let this trust grow with each breath, deepening your connection to your inner strength.*

Part 3: Responsibility and Accomplishment

> *Now, breathe into the words "responsibility" and "accomplishment." Imagine these*

> qualities merging with the light in your root chakra. Feel a sense of purpose and readiness to take on responsibilities and achieve your soul's mission in your own unique way.
> - Reflect on your potential to serve and accomplish. Breathe into the feeling that you are meant for something important, even if you're not sure what it is yet. Allow this sense of knowing to grow within you.

Part 4: Embracing Your Inner Throne

> - Imagine a magnificent, golden throne in front of you. Use your imagination to see all the details: its shape, size, and any intricate carvings or simple designs. If visualizing is challenging, use your other senses—how does it feel to the touch? Is it warm or cool? This throne is a **majestic symbol of your inner sovereignty and power and is for you and you only.**
> - Approach your throne and, when you're ready, take your seat. Feel the support and strength of the throne beneath you. As you sit, recognize that this throne represents your place of power and purpose in your life.
> - Breathe into the sense of ownership. Allow yourself to feel a deep, inner knowing that you have an important role to fulfill. Embrace and breathe into all the feelings this brings up in you. Don't judge them. You are safe to feel everything from fear or apprehension to joy, power or ecstasy.

This meditation is about connecting with your root chakra and embracing your sense of inner power. There's no need to set goals or uncover your life's purpose right now. Instead, focus on feeling grounded, secure, and ready for whatever lies ahead.

Remember, healing and empowerment are ongoing journeys. Be patient with yourself as you continue to grow and evolve. You are exactly where you need to be at this moment.

Thank you for doing this meditation. Take a few more deep breaths, and when you're ready, gently open your eyes. Carry this sense of grounding and purpose with you throughout your day.

Feel free to revisit this meditation whenever you need to reconnect with your root chakra and your sense of inner power.

Testimonial: It was the second gathering of the program. My life had been turned upside down with the Alzheimer's death of a 41 year partner, a cancer death of my beloved sister, and the cancer deaths of two dear friends—all within a 2 year period. I was exhausted, from continuous caregiving, from loss and grief, and taking care of myself as best I could with the help of good friends. Before this season of grief, I was full of energy each morning, heading into my day for work I loved, and life that was purposeful. Now I dreaded putting my feet over the edge of the bed each day, to find myself aching with fatigue, weak, and not looking for anything beyond surviving the present moment. My spiritual life has always been important to me, and I felt enough support from those embodied in this physical life as well as those who had left to keep going. I had asked the Universe to take me deeper into my spiritual life during the journey of grief over those two prior years, and an important part of that was finding Cheryl and beginning the work of healing old wounds. I made the decision after some of this work to take the advanced Higher State Throat Chakra program which included the Throne work.

In this Taking a Seat in the Throne session, we were invited to take our place in a seat of empowerment, particularly as women. I was moved to a new level, literally and figuratively. I felt my spirit and energy rise into the throne, felt an old, familiar part of myself come back into my being, and knew on this level that I have strength and power. As anyone who has gone through the journey of grief knows, exhaustion can be a regular and often discouraging visitor. When I come back to my throne, I feel myself filled with energy, at least for the moment, and know all will be well. I am powerful again. My throne is made of multi-colored light, located in a cave that is filled with a golden glow, and open to the skies above. It is my spiritual home now, as I move forward in my journey to heal and grow into my power again, making another new beginning.

As we conclude this chapter, remember that taking your seat is about more than just embracing your soul's mission; it's about stepping into your inherent power and owning your place in the world. Embrace your unique gifts, trust in your journey, and allow yourself to grow beyond mere stability. Your throne symbolizes your innate wisdom and strength. By claiming it, you pave the way for profound personal and spiritual transformation. Believe in the beauty of your dreams, and let this chapter be a reminder that you are destined for greatness. Now is the time to take your seat and shine your light into the world.

17

Use Your Struggles to Catapult to a Higher State of Being

"Out of difficulties grow miracles."
— *Jean de La Bruyère*

You have read about energy patterns and subconscious blocks in previous chapters. My goal here is to add depth to that understanding by exploring how to use your struggles as catalysts for reaching a higher state of being.

Negative energy patterns, often manifesting as negative self-talk, originate from past traumas and unmet needs during childhood. These early experiences shape the energetic imprints that influence your self-perception and how you handle life's challenges. Try reflecting on childhood moments when you didn't receive the emotional support you needed then. Note how those experiences may have ingrained critical energy patterns, pushing you to meet external expectations as a survival mechanism. Like most of us, as an adult, these patterns might still resonate within you, echoing doubts and fears, and trying to protect you from perceived threats. While they aim to safeguard you, these patterns or behaviors will block you from realizing your full potential.

Many of my clients have experienced emotional neglect in early childhood. This doesn't necessarily mean they had terrible parents, rather, most parents simply didn't know how to be the emotional resources their children needed. Parents didn't receive it for themselves as children. It is a fundamental human need to have our emotions acknowledged and validated. As children and even as adults, we need to be comforted. When we don't get this support, it affects our brain development.

Research indicates that emotional neglect can especially harm the frontal cortex, the area responsible for planning, decision-making, and memory (Perry, 2002; DeBellis, 2005). The National Institutes of Health (NIH) also notes that emotional neglect is associated with smaller hippocampal volumes. Patients with major depressive disorder (MDD) who experienced childhood emotional neglect often have smaller left hippocampal white matter volumes compared to those who didn't experience such neglect. Despite the impacts of early emotional neglect on brain development, the brain's inherent neuroplasticity offers hope for transformation. Neuroplasticity is the brain's ability to reorganize itself by forming new neural connections throughout life. The energy healing and empowerment techniques in this book can harness this ability of your brain to rewire old energy patterns shaped by past neglect.

Another area to take a look at is resentments. Do you hold any resentments toward anyone? Brene Brown states in her book "Dare to Lead," "wherever there is resentment, there is a boundary issue." Harboring resentment can be tempting because it gives a false sense of power and control. It provides energy and motivation to get things done and also helps us avoid uncomfortable conversations. It offers a feeling of safety by protecting us from vulnerability and allows us to feel "right." Resentment can make others feel guilty. It helps us to avoid dealing with deeper feelings beneath the anger. It also allows us to hold onto a relationship that might otherwise end and lets us avoid responsibility by staying in the role of the victim.

Many say that forgiveness is the answer, and I agree, but most people don't know how to truly forgive. When I do chakra readings, I almost always see a certain amount of wounds of betrayal. I see this dark energy at the back of the heart chakra. Some people will say, "I've done a lot of forgiveness, so why is this energy still there?" Those people usually forgive at the level of the mind and stuff their resentments deep into their subconscious. When someone shows up with light at the back of the heart chakra, I can tell they have an excellent grasp of true or complete forgiveness and have practiced it.

To forgive fully, remember that the deeper the wounding, the longer the forgiveness process. We must process our own feelings first so that we can see the other in a different light. This often gives us compassion for the other. Even horrific events like sexual abuse can be completely forgiven. I encourage you to reflect or journal on your resentments and bring them into the ACE Method to be healed.

> *"As smoking is to the lungs, so is resentment to the soul;*
>
> *even one puff is bad for you."*
>
> — *Elizabeth Gilbert*

Let's dive in here and harness the brain's neuroplasticity to reprogram old patterns and create positive new pathways. I invite you to use the ACE method described earlier in this book to access the emotions that are still trapped in your subconscious.

Advanced ACE Method Meditation

You can begin by looking at a particular situation in your life that is not working for you in one way or another. Start with the number one emotion that comes up when you think about the situation. Breathe into that emotion and then go deeper, asking yourself "What is the deeper emotion underneath?". Go as deep as you can in this access stage.

You want to keep going until you get to the deepest emotion and then follow that emotion back to early childhood. Ask your subconscious "When did this begin?" And let yourself go back to the time that it started. Let your body answer for you. Keep breathing fully so you stay in your right brain. If you start thinking continuous thoughts, that is a sign you are in the left brain and won't get there that way. Check your breath as this often happens when we stop breathing fully. It's totally normal and it's okay if that happens; just breathe fully and go back to breathing into the emotion and wherever you left off. You can trust your subconscious to help you.

Once you have breathed into all the emotions held in your subconscious, ask yourself "What subconscious beliefs do I have about myself, people, and the world?", and wait for the answers. You can also finish one or all of these sentences:

- I am _____
- People are _____
- Life is _____
- To survive, I have to_____
- To be loved, I must _____
- I hold resentments toward _____
- Add in any subconscious belief which created an unhealthy attitude, behavior, or way of coping.

ALL your answers are inside you! Once you breathe into all the emotions from early childhood, thereby clearing them, you can continue with the reparenting until your younger self feels a number of much more uplifting emotions. Help her/him breathe into those new emotions as described in the ACE Method.

Once your younger self is feeling loved, valued, and other warm and fuzzy emotions, imagine holding her in your root chakra (or whatever chakra you are *working on), letting her know you will return. Continue with the Full Breath and ask yourself questions like:*

- *How has that block or wound served me?*
- *How did it help me grow?*
- *What quality am I meant to develop through this? Use the difficult emotions I felt to understand. Ie: unworthiness helps you build the muscles to overcome it and live your life from a place of self worth. Growing up feeling powerless helps you grow into your most powerful self.*
- *How do the answers to the above questions affect your purpose in life?*
- *Complete the sentence: In order to become/accomplish/live/have _____, I need to _____. What is your deepest truth here? Keep breathing fully and let this all come out of your subconscious, not your left brain. You will be surprised and elated.*

Doing this work involves acknowledging your worth and validating your emotions throughout the practice. Practicing self-compassion during your energy healing sessions will create more self-compassion throughout your life. Practicing self-compassion means treating yourself with kindness during moments of failure or suffering and lovingly honoring all your emotions without judgment. This self-kindness helps neutralize the negative energy from past neglect and fosters a nurturing, healing inner energy field.

I invite you to open up to taking the Full Breath to the next level. Once in meditation for sometime,

> *especially during the empowerment phase, allow yourself to be breathed.*

You're probably asking, "what does it mean to allow yourself to be breathed?". Let me explain. You've opened up to receiving at a greater level, surrendered to being held by the whole Universe, and now, you can move to the greatest level of the Full Breath, opening up and allowing yourself to be breathed by the Universe. It's not you who is doing the breathing, you are receiving, one with the Universe.

> *In the beginning, it's challenging to fully open up to this practice so you may use your mind and imagination to focus on the technique. On every exhale, imagine you are being inhaled by the Universe and on every exhale, you are being exhaled by the Universe. Open up to being breathed. Surrender and allow yourself to be breathed.*

By surrendering to being breathed by the Universe, you experience a deep state of relaxation. This reduces stress and promotes overall well-being. It also facilitates the release of deep and long trapped emotions, leading to profound emotional healing and balance. This practice deepens your connection to the divine, fostering a sense of oneness with the Universe, and as you align with the rhythm of the Universe, so you tap into a limitless source of energy, enhancing your vitality and zest for life. By embracing this practice, you cultivate a sense of empowerment and confidence, knowing you are supported by a higher power.

As you go through your process, seek out relationships and support networks where your emotions are acknowledged and validated. Let a close friend or family member know what you are working on and ask for support. Ask if it's okay if you stay in closer touch so you can share your changes. This can empower you to break free from old energy patterns of not feeling supported and connected. Empathic interactions nurture a supportive energy field that fosters healing and growth.

In addition to the ACE Method, you can further integrate your healing and empowerment process by engaging in creative activities such as art, dance, or writing, which can also provide an outlet for processing and transforming negative energy into positive energy. This creative flow empowers you to harness your newly discovered inner strengths and talents.

Practice heartful reflection by regularly tuning into your heart in an inquiring way and reflect on your progress with compassion, unconditional self-love, and gratitude. Use the Full Breath while you reflect to lock this into your subconscious. Recognize and celebrate your achievements, no matter how small. This reflective practice solidifies new, empowering energy patterns and promotes ongoing growth. It would also be beneficial to journal about your process, your progress, and your achievements.

As you undergo internal shifts and realign your energy patterns, it becomes crucial to express these changes in all areas of your life. Naturally, this process involves setting healthy boundaries, which are vital for reinforcing positive energy patterns and promoting self-growth. Boundaries act as a reflection of your newfound self-awareness and inner strength, allowing you to protect your personal space and maintain the positive transformations you've achieved. By clearly articulating and upholding these boundaries, you honor your needs and values, creating a balanced flow of energy in your interactions. This not only preserves your emotional and mental well-being but also supports your ongoing self-development. Embracing these boundaries enables you to focus on your own goals and aspirations with renewed confidence, ensuring that your external environment aligns with your internal growth and contributes to a harmonious, fulfilling life.

Pay attention to procrastination. Procrastination is an energy management issue, not a time management issue. Procrastination often becomes a method to manage the discomfort tied to stress and the fear of failure. You might delay tasks until the pressure builds, convincing yourself that the last-minute energy surge enhances your performance. In reality, this reinforces a false belief—that your energy aligns with the "unsuccessful" pattern. Procrastination creates a deceptive sense of safety, shielding you from the energy shifts associated with failure or success.

Viewing procrastination as a time management problem misses the root cause. Procrastination is actually about managing your energy, not your schedule. You're not avoiding the task itself but the negative energy associated with it, such as fear of failure, anxiety, or inadequacy. Imagine having a significant project. Instead of starting, you feel overwhelmed by a low-energy state of dread and inadequacy, leading you to delay the task. Procrastination offers a brief escape from these negative energy patterns but doesn't address the deeper energetic issue.

> To break free from procrastination, reframe how you perceive your tasks. Focus on their deeper energetic value and significance rather than the discomfort they bring. Reflect on these questions:
>
> - Why does this task hold an energetic value for me?
> - How does it contribute to my energetic growth?
> - What can I learn about my energy patterns through completing it?

By viewing tasks as opportunities for energetic growth and self-discovery, you can evoke positive energy that motivates you to act. This shift transforms challenges into pathways for personal and spiritual expansion. To avoid procrastination, it's crucial to discern which tasks are truly worth doing and which are not. Once you have this clarity, you can make decisions with confidence and follow through. Remember, it's okay to let go of certain tasks and prioritize what truly matters.

Cultivating compassion and forgiveness toward yourself is crucial in overcoming procrastination and negative energy patterns. Recognize that procrastination isn't about laziness or inefficiency; it's about grappling with deeper energetic issues. Welcome all aspects of your energy, even those parts that procrastinate. Understand that these behaviors are coping mechanisms within your energy field, and it's okay to struggle. By extending compassion and forgiveness to yourself, you create a nurturing energetic space that encourages action rather than avoidance.

To truly progress, shift from asking "why" questions, which can lead to self-criticism, to "what" questions that inspire energetic growth and action. Instead of pondering, "Why am I procrastinating?" ask, "What can I do right now to shift my energy forward?" And, my favorite, "What is it I don't want to feel right now?" Feel whatever emotion is getting in the way through meditation with the Full Breath and let it move. What is it that wants to be felt? Inspiration, excitement? This change in questioning and clearing any block focuses you on constructive energy actions rather than self-blame. Instead of dwelling on why you haven't started a task, think about what small energetic step you can take immediately. This approach reduces the emotional and energetic burden and helps build positive momentum in your energy field.

Every challenge or struggle you face is a divine opportunity for energetic growth. the Universe supports you continuously, offering each difficulty as a chance to develop new energetic skills and uncover your inner energetic superpowers.

> *When you encounter a challenge, resist the urge to complain, blame, or flee. Instead, ask yourself:*
> - *How is this challenge serving my personal/spiritual growth?*
> - *What lesson does this problem reflect in my energy field that I need to learn?*

By viewing struggles as opportunities for personal and spiritual development in your energy field, you can transform problems into powerful catalysts for energetic growth. This reflective approach helps you uncover hidden strengths and insights within your energy patterns, propelling you to a higher energetic state.

The Universe's energetic support is always present, guiding you through struggles and nurturing your energetic growth. Each challenge is a divine energetic lesson designed to elevate you, even if it doesn't feel that way. Embrace this cosmic energetic support by trusting that every difficulty contains the seeds of your energetic advancement. When you face a problem, instead of seeing it as an obstacle, view it as a personalized energetic growth opportunity from the Universe. This perspective allows you to approach challenges with curiosity and openness, ready to uncover the energetic wisdom they hold.

By understanding and addressing the root causes of your negative energy patterns and procrastination, and by embracing challenges as opportunities for energetic growth, you can become your own energy worker. This spiritual journey involves recognizing how your past shapes your present energy, transforming your relationship with stress and tasks, and fostering self-compassion in your energy field. Harness your struggles as catalysts for personal and spiritual growth in your energy. Realign your energy patterns and elevate yourself to a higher state of being. Embrace your path with patience, kindness, and trust in the Universe, knowing that each step forward is a triumph in becoming the best energetic version of yourself.

> *Pause and ask yourself, amidst negative energy patterns or procrastination:*
>
> - *What is it that's hard to feel energetically?*
> - *What is it that I am resisting.*
> - *What energy is currently not in alignment with me?*
> - *How do I feel this in my body?*
>
> *Embrace these feelings with compassion and curiosity, for they hold the keys to your energetic growth and transformation.*

Incorporating gratitude into your journey of transformation is a profound way to enhance your progress and deepen your healing. It's important to recognize that forced gratitude isn't as authentic as gratitude that is felt naturally. When you genuinely feel the support of another human, your spirit guides, or the whole Universe, you can catch gratitude wanting to flow through you. This kind of gratitude arises spontaneously and authentically, providing a sense of nourishment and connection.

You may find yourself entering into a state of gratitude for certain wounds and traumas that you have suffered because they served you in becoming stronger and ultimately more powerful in your life. Embracing gratitude for these challenges allows you to see them as catalysts for growth and empowerment rather than mere obstacles. It's through overcoming these difficulties that you will be able to access deeper layers of your authentic self and unlock your true potential.

The power of love flowing through you in gratitude is transformative. When you open yourself up to this flow, you allow love and gratitude to permeate every aspect of your being. This creates a positive feedback loop, where the more gratitude you feel, the more love and support you attract from the Universe. This loving energy not only heals but also elevates you, enabling you to live more fully and authentically. Embracing this state of gratitude transforms your struggles into opportunities for growth, reinforcing the idea that every challenge you face is a step toward becoming your true, powerful self.

As you reach the end of this chapter, remember that your struggles are not just obstacles—they are opportunities to propel you into a higher state of being and to tap into your authentic power and open up more and more to the power of the Universe flowing through you. Every challenge you face holds the potential for deep transformation, offering you the chance to rewire old energy patterns, heal past wounds, and embrace new, empowering beliefs. By viewing your difficulties through the lens of growth and transformation, you turn them into catalysts for discovering your true self and aligning with your highest purpose. Embrace these moments, for they are the very crucible in which your most powerful self is forged. Trust in the process, knowing that each struggle is a step toward the much more amazing and authentically powerful person you are destined to become.

18
From Blocked to Powerful - Summary

"What you seek is seeking you."
— *Rumi*

You have read about energy patterns and subconscious blocks in previous chapters. My goal here is to add depth to that understanding by exploring how to use your struggles as catalysts for reaching a higher state of being.

As we reach the end of this journey, let's take a moment to reflect on everything you've learned and accomplished. You've embarked on an adventure of healing and empowerment, explored your inner world, and discovered the tools to transform from blocked to powerful. Throughout this book, you've gained insights and techniques to clear your blocks, find clarity, and step into your true power. Each chapter has provided you with a piece of the puzzle, guiding you toward a more fulfilled and empowered life.

In **Chapter 1: Understanding Subconscious Blocks**, you laid the foundation by recognizing the unseen forces that hold you back. This awareness was the first step in your journey toward healing and empowerment. Understanding these blocks allowed you to see how they affect your daily life and provided the motivation to start clearing them.

In **Chapter 2: Authentic Power**, we explored the concept of power, particularly the challenges women face in embracing their true power. Understanding that it's not about you but about allowing the Universe to move through you can liberate you from the constraints of the ego and align you with a higher purpose. You learned that true power comes from within and is about authenticity and alignment with your soul's purpose.

In **Chapter 3: Embracing Discovery and Change**, you learned the importance of being open to new experiences and the transformative power of change. This chapter set the stage for your journey of self-discovery, encouraging you to embrace change as a constant and beneficial part of life.

Chapter 4: How I Cleared My Blocks, Gained Clarity, and Started Living My Purpose (The First Time) provided a personal narrative of my journey, illustrating how clearing blocks and gaining clarity can lead to living your true purpose. I hope my story has inspired you to embark on your own path of self-discovery and empowerment.

In **Chapter 5: First Step to Becoming Your Own Energy Worker**, you took the initial steps to harness your inner energy, beginning to clear the blocks that have held you back. This chapter gave you practical tools for you to start working with your inner energy and understanding its impact on your life.

Chapter 6: Accessing and Clearing Subconscious Blocks, equipped you with practical techniques to dive deep into your subconscious, identifying and clearing the obstacles that prevent you from reaching your full potential. This chapter was pivotal in helping you understand the root causes of your blocks and how to address them effectively.

In **Chapter 7: Empowerment - Reprogramming the Subconscious**, you learned how to rewire your subconscious mind, replacing limiting beliefs with empowering ones to support your journey toward true empowerment. This chapter provided you with tools to transform your internal dialogue and create a supportive inner environment.

Chapter 8: Developing Receptivity focused on opening yourself up to receive guidance, support, and blessings from the Universe. This chapter emphasized the importance of being receptive to the flow of life and how this openness can lead to greater clarity and support.

Chapter 9: Are You a Hole Filler? challenged you to look deeper into your behaviors and patterns, helping you recognize the ways in which you might be filling emotional voids rather than addressing their root causes. This chapter encouraged you to find healthier ways to fulfill your emotional needs.

Chapter 10: New Beginnings encouraged you to embrace change and recognize the moments of clarity that guide you toward your soul's purpose. This chapter reinforced the idea that every ending is a new beginning and provided strategies for navigating transitions.

Chapter 11: Healing and Empowerment to True Purpose highlighted the connection between healing and finding your true purpose, reinforcing the idea that empowerment comes from within. This chapter helped you see how healing your past can open up new possibilities for your future.

Chapter 12: Spike of Purpose inspired you to harness moments of clarity and purpose, using them as a driving force for your journey. This chapter emphasized the importance of recognizing and acting on moments of inspiration.

In **Chapter 13: Clearing Blocks in Your Environment**, you discovered how your surroundings influence your inner state. By clearing physical clutter and creating a harmonious environment, you support your internal healing and empowerment. This chapter highlighted the connection between our external space and internal well-being.

Chapter 14: Evolving Through Heart-Centered Shamanism taught you the value of connecting deeply with yourself and the natural world to uncover profound wisdom and healing. This practice taught you to trust your inner guidance and embrace the interconnectedness of all life. You learned how ancient shamanic practices can be integrated into modern life to facilitate deep healing.

In **Chapter 15: Take Your Seat**, you learned to own your power and take your rightful place in the world, embodying the lessons and insights you've gained throughout this journey. This chapter encouraged you to step into your authority and live your truth with confidence.

Chapter 16: Use Your Struggles to Catapult to a Higher State of Being showed you how every struggle can be a stepping stone toward greater resilience and wisdom. You now understand that challenges are opportunities for growth and transformation. This chapter provided strategies for turning adversity into advantage.

As you close this book, remember that this is not the end but a new beginning. You are now equipped with the knowledge, tools, and confidence to continue your journey from blocked to powerful. Your path is uniquely yours, and every step you take is a testament to your strength and resilience.

If at any point you feel uncertain or need additional support, remember that you don't have to do it all on your own. Consider scheduling a chakra reading with me or an Insight Session to gain more personalized insights and guidance. These sessions can help you clear any remaining blocks and provide you with the clarity you need to move forward.

You are destined for greatness. Embrace your journey with an open heart, knowing that every challenge is an opportunity for growth and every victory is a stepping stone toward your highest self. As you move forward, let your light shine brightly, inspiring others to embark on their own journeys of healing and empowerment.

Remember my quote in the beginning. Please receive me saying it to you here:

Breathe in: "You are Powerful Beyond Belief, Powerful Beyond What You Can Imagine."

And event take the next step and make it your own mantra to practice on the full breath:

> *I am powerful beyond belief, powerful beyond what I can imagine.*

It has been such an honor to be a part of your transformative journey. Remember, you are powerful, you are worthy, you matter so much and you are destined for greatness. Continue to break through your blocks, discover your clarity, and live your soul's purpose with unwavering faith and courage.

With love and light,
Cheryl

19
Thank You

"Silent gratitude isn't much use to anyone"

— *Gertrude Stein*

Writing this book has been an incredible journey, and it would not have been possible without the support, encouragement, and inspiration from the Universe and so many remarkable individuals.

First and foremost, I extend my deepest gratitude to the Universe for its persistent, loving nudges, guiding me to write this third book. I never imagined undertaking this journey until I started receiving these divine signals. I am profoundly thankful for the unending spiritual support every step of the way, helping me sort and filter through what the Universe intended to be written through me and what was not meant for this book. Your constant presence helped me breathe through the emotions and process my own blocks, allowing me to share everything in these pages.

Thank you, my beloved John, for your unwavering love and endless support, and for always standing by my side. To my children, your joy and curiosity inspire me daily.

To my friends, thank you for your understanding, patience, and encouragement throughout this process. Your words of wisdom and moments of laughter have kept me grounded and motivated.

I am immensely grateful to my clients and students. Your courage, trust, and commitment to your own growth and transformation have been a constant source of inspiration. You are the reason I do what I do, and it is an honor to be part of your journey.

A heartfelt thank you to my editors and publishing team. Your expertise, guidance, and hard work have brought this book to life. Your belief in my vision and your dedication to excellence have made this project a reality.

To all my mentors and teachers, both named and unnamed, thank you for sharing your wisdom and for guiding me on my path. Your teachings have shaped my understanding and practice of healing and empowerment.

I would also like to acknowledge the countless individuals whose work and words have inspired me along the way. Your contributions to the fields of spirituality, healing, and personal development have enriched my own journey and informed the pages of this book.

Finally, to you, the reader, thank you for picking up this book. I hope it serves as a source of inspiration, profound insight, and empowerment on your journey. May you find the courage to clear your subconscious blocks, uncover your deepest truths, and awaken your inner power, living a life of profound fulfillment.

Writing this book has been an incredible journey, and it would not have been possible without the support, encouragement, and inspiration from so many remarkable individuals.

First and foremost, I extend my deepest gratitude to the Universe for guiding me to write yet another book, and helping me get out of the way throughout the process.

Thank you my beloved John, for your unwavering love and endless support and for always standing by my side. To my children, your joy and curiosity inspire me daily.

To my friends, thank you for your understanding, patience, and encouragement throughout this process. Your words of wisdom and moments of laughter have kept me grounded and motivated.

I am immensely grateful to my clients and students. Your courage, trust, and commitment to your own growth and transformation have been a constant source of inspiration. You are the reason I do what I do, and it is an honor to be part of your journey.

A heartfelt thank you to my editors and publishing team. Your expertise, guidance, and hard work have brought this book to life. Your belief in my vision and your dedication to excellence have made this project a reality.

To all my mentors and teachers, both named and unnamed, thank you for sharing your wisdom and for guiding me on my path. Your teachings have shaped my understanding and practice of healing and empowerment.

I would also like to acknowledge the countless individuals whose work and words have inspired me along the way. Your contributions to the fields of spirituality, healing, and personal development have enriched my own journey and informed the pages of this book.

Finally, to you, the reader, thank you for picking up this book. I hope it has served as a source of inspiration, profound insight, and transformational healing and empowerment on your journey. May you find the courage to clear your subconscious blocks, uncover your deepest truths, and awaken your authentic power, living a life of profound fulfillment.

You've taken significant steps toward unlocking your true potential and allowing the power of the Universe to flow through you. But your journey doesn't end here—it's just the beginning.

If you're feeling inspired and ready to dive deeper, I invite you to take the next step with me. For those ready to go further, my Insight Sessions are designed to provide you with tailored guidance and support. Together, we will explore the specific challenges you're facing, look at clearing any remaining blocks, and empower you to move forward with confidence and clarity.

Schedule Your Insight Session

Just click the link or scan the QR code:

https://cherylstelte.kartra.com/calendar/discoverycall

As you continue on this path of transformation, remember that every step forward is a testament to your strength and resilience. Trust in the journey ahead, knowing that the Universe is guiding you toward a life filled with purpose, joy, and limitless possibilities. Your future is bright, and you are more powerful than you can imagine.

About the Author

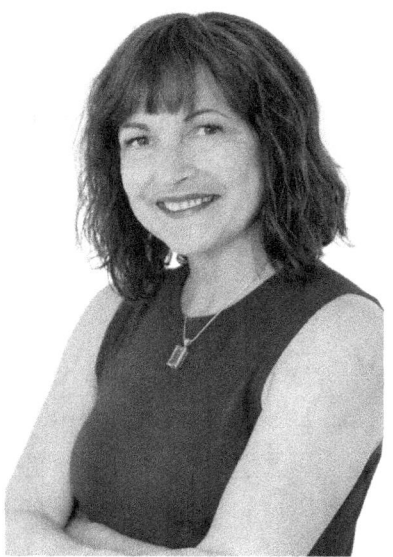

With a rich three-decade journey as a Spiritual Entrepreneur, Cheryl Stelte has illuminated the paths of numerous individuals as a respected spiritual coach, master healer, bestselling author, and engaging speaker. Her unwavering dedication revolves around empowering women who know they are meant for more, guiding them to clear their subconscious blocks, gain the clarity they want, and ultimately become their most powerful selves, beyond what they could imagine.

Through Cheryl's compassionate guidance, clients undergo profound transformations, achieving milestones once thought unattainable. Cheryl's dedication to women's empowerment began in her first business in Fashion Design and later Stelte Design, Designing for the Soul, where she fostered new skills and confidence in staff. She helped clients discover their true selves through Interior Design, Spiritual Readings, Remodeling, Energy Clearings, and Remodeling. Her adventurous spirit has led her to reside with the Maasai in Kenya and help stop early forced marriage and forced genital mutilation. and the Shuar in Ecuador, where she again taught women new skills, fostering self assurance.

Cheryl holds diplomas in acupressure (Cdn. Acupressure College), fashion design (Blanche MacDonald); interior design (Victoria, BC), elemental space clearing (Denise Linn), hatha yoga Instructor (India), reiki master (India), and shamanic trainings (Foundation for Shamanic Studies & Claude Poncelet). Cheryl received certifications from IAMHeart as a spiritual mentor, coach, personal retreat guide, and Hurqalya Healing Practitioner.

As the visionary force behind the Star of Divine Light Institute and the innovative creator of the Azarias Energy Healing Certification Program, Cheryl empowers coaches, and entrepreneurs with potent tools for catalyzing transformative shifts in their clients.

Cheryl is a Canadian living in the Rocky Mountains of Colorado with her husband John. She has two wonderful adult children, two grandchildren and enjoys hiking, kayaking, traveling, cooking and most of all, helping women ignite their inner power.

References

1. Goyal, M., et al. (2014). "Meditation Programs for Psychological Stress and Well-being: A Systematic Review and Meta-analysis." JAMA Internal Medicine. Link
2. Bushell, W. C., et al. (2009). "Meditation and Neuroplasticity: Current Evidence and Future Directions." Annals of the New York Academy of Sciences. Link
3. Critchley, H. D., & Garfinkel, S. N. (2017). "Interoception and Emotion." Current Opinion in Psychology. Link
4. Porges, S. W. (2011). "The Polyvagal Theory: Neurophysiological Foundations of Emotions, Attachment, Communication, and Self-regulation." W. W. Norton & Company. Link
5. Lutz, A., et al. (2008). "Attention Regulation and Monitoring in Meditation." Trends in Cognitive Sciences. Link

FROM BLOCKED TO POWERFUL

FROM BLOCKED TO POWERFUL

FROM BLOCKED TO POWERFUL

www.ingramcontent.com/pod-product-compliance
Lightning Source LLC
Chambersburg PA
CBHW071828210526
45479CB00001B/35